The Essential Oils Companion for Mindfulness

Heather Godfrey

This is a First Edition of the paperback
The Essential Oils Companion for Mindfulness
Copyright © 2016 Heather Godfrey
ISBN: 978-1-910094-02-0
Published March 2016
By Magic Oxygen
www.MagicOxygen.co.uk
editor@MagicOxygen.co.uk
Heather Godfrey has asserted her right under the
Copyright, Designs and Patents Act 1988
to be identified as the author of this work.
Edited by Izzy Robertson
A catalogue record for this book is available from
the British Library.

Printed by Lightning Source UK Ltd; committed to improving environmental performance by driving down emissions and reducing, reusing and recycling waste.
View their eco-policy at www.LightningSource.com
Set in 12pt Arial
Titles: Courgette

So far as may legally and effectively be provided, no liability of any kind or nature whatsoever, whether in negligence, under statute, or otherwise, is accepted by the author or the publishers for the accuracy or safety of any of the information or advice contained in, or in any way relating to, any part of the content of this book.

The information provided in the following chapters is not presented as an alternative or substitute for professional advice or healthcare.

The aim of this book is to provide a complementary preventative tool to support wellness and wellbeing.

Contents

Acknowledgements

My sincere thanks and gratitude are extended to April Tatlock, Jane Logie, my Godmother May Copp, Linda Manzioni and Sonraya Grace for their unconditional support, belief and encouragement, and to Izzy Robertson for patiently scrolling through every word in her editing quest.

Photographs featured in this book were taken with kind permission at Compton Acres Gardens (Poole, Dorset, UK BH13 7ES www.comptonacres.co.uk); my thanks and appreciation are extended to Joseph Googan, gardener, for sharing his wealth of knowledge and expertise. Examples of essential oil bearing plants (along with many other herbaceous and medicinal plants) located within the gardens include: angelica (Angelica officinalis), cypress (Cupressus sempervirens), fennel (Foeniculum vulgare), mint (Mentha piperita), pine (Pinus sylvestris), rose (Rosa centifolia) and rosemary (Rosmarinus officinalis).

Essential oils and vegetable oils which appear in the photographs were supplied by NHR Organic Oils, Brighton, Sussex, UK BH1 5TN (www.nhrorganicoils.com), Oshadhi Organic and Wildcrafted Essential Oils, Cambridge, UK (www.oshadhi.co.uk), Tisserand Aromatherapy, West Sussex, UK BN6 9LS (www.tisserand.com), The Frankincense Store, London, UK NW1 8AH (www.freeyoursenses.co.uk), Base Formula Limited, Melton Mowbray, Leicestershire, UK LE13 0RG (www.baseformula.com). Please also note that when not being photographed or used, the essential oils featured are kept inside closed containers, which protect them from UV light, and are stored in a fridge to keep them cool.

Preface

I was introduced to essential oils many years ago, when I worked for Robert Tisserand in London, during those early days when he first began developing his business. Then, I was a teenager, naïve and idealistic, believing that I had so many years ahead, my life spreading out before me with endless possibility. So, when a friend beckoned me to join her in Corsica to work for a season, I went without hesitation, assuming I could simply pick up the threads when I was ready to return. Within a year, however, I was married and expecting my first child, my path decided and etched to a distant horizon. Serendipitously one day, four beautiful children and some years later, I found myself in a bookshop, waiting for a friend.

Browsing the shelves in front of me, I noticed with pleasant surprise a book written by Robert, "The Art of Aromatherapy". Intrigued, I flicked through the pages. Memories instantly flooded through me; the air I breathed seemed suddenly imbued with the scent of rose, ylang ylang and chamomile, as I recalled, as if only the day before, Robert, Jonathon ('Jack' and 'Hans', as they were known then) and me weighing dried chamomile and rose flowers and packing small brown bottles of essential oils. I remembered the indulgent ambiance the scents created: the sweet; the spicy; the earthy; the leafy; the fruity; the woody; the floral; the deeply rich, the playfully light – exuding, permeating every corner of the space, dispelling the dank background smell in the small old building we occupied then. From that chance moment in the bookshop, revisiting the comfort, the familiarity, the tingle of excitement I felt, my inspiration was rekindled; my children growing, it was time to pick up the threads I had started to weave, to complete the journey I began during those early years in London.

I continue to this day to be inspired and intrigued by the psycho-emotional support essential oils offer, their ability to uplift, brace and 'ground' among many other significant qualities; simple, yet important when dealing with 'everyday' life. Of course, I am aware at my age, that there is no magic formula, that life is a journey and we each travel on our own path, which may sometimes be easy, sometimes difficult to tread. However, there are positive and negative ways of coping with the stresses and joys of everyday life. Essential oils appear to be a multidynamic gift presented by nature, offered, it seems, to accompany our journey through life, through the ups and downs, the joys and challenges, like a supportive friend.

Through my clinical practice, observing my clients response to essential oils, and through my own experience, I notice how enriching this relationship is, practical and pleasurable, healing and uplifting, and how this in turn, may also translate into a healthy sense of wellbeing.

Viewed through the lens of several years' professional experience working with clients and students, Aromantique 'The Essence of Wellness' incorporates a series of books written to support those who want to use essential oils to enhance their wellbeing. Collectively these books present an introductory yet informative self-help guide that will support the practical and safe use of essential oils, while also providing a sound foundation for the prospective student to build their repertoire.

I have had the fortune to work with a range of clients (parents, grandparents, carers supporting others, teachers, researchers, managers, nurses, acupuncturists, counsellors and a variety of healthcare professionals amongst others) who have sought treatments for many different reasons. These include balancing physical and psycho-emotional wellbeing while working in demanding roles; managing stress or a stress related condition, such as insomnia, mild depression or anxiety; as support during challenging life-events such as bereavement, redundancy or relationship breakdown and, conversely, exciting events such as moving house, changing jobs or getting married. Sometimes it is for the simple but possibly most significant reason of all, to relax and enhance a sense of wellbeing. Indeed, inspiration for the Aromantique compilation evolved from observing my clients' response to the scent of essential oils. I observed how the experience of odour absorption and perception drew their attention and awareness, all-be-it fleetingly, into the moment; also noticing how those moments were enriched as the odour permeated their psychic 'being' and appeared to trigger a psycho-emotional response and effect. These responses were initially observed through a softening of facial expression and calmer breathing, after which clients reported their experience of increased energy, clearer thinking and a sense of feeling relaxed and 'grounded'. There is also a physiological response via the nervous system.

Essential Oils

There are hundreds of essential oils available to purchase 'over the counter' or through mail order. However, not all are suitable for personal use. Essential oils are mainly produced for the pharmaceutical, food and manufacturing, perfume and cosmetic industries. Indeed, the aromatherapy market accounts for less than 5% of the total overall quantity of essential oils produced. A select but significant complementary group of essential oils is presented here to provide a foundation on which to safely build your repertoire. This specific group of essential oils was originally purposefully derived to apply in the context of special needs, working with vulnerable and/or sensitive clients, and includes some of the potentially least hazardous (although no essential oil is completely hazard-free) yet still very effective essences. Collectively referred to as 'Essential Oil Gems', they cover a valuable spectrum of therapeutic properties pertinent for those wishing to use essential oils as self-help remedies and for the discerning student to apply as a sound foundation for learning. In order to help contextualize their properties, however, the information presented here includes a wide range of essential oils. 'Essential Oil Gems' are highlighted amongst these for ease of identification and are covered in most depth. For more details regarding the other essential oils, please go to the Aromantique website.

Essential oils are effective when used individually, but their effects may potentially increase when carefully blended together. As well as observing their chemical and therapeutic properties, the sensual, odorous quality of essential oils lends pleasure and expressive creativity to the 'art of blending' (Tisserand 1997). So in this sense odour, like colour, can be applied to 'paint a picture', create ambiance, express and enhance feelings, emotions and moods, while at the same time providing valuable immunological support.

The information provided in the following chapters is not presented as an alternative or substitute for professional advice or healthcare. The aim of this book is to provide a complementary preventative tool to support wellness and wellbeing.

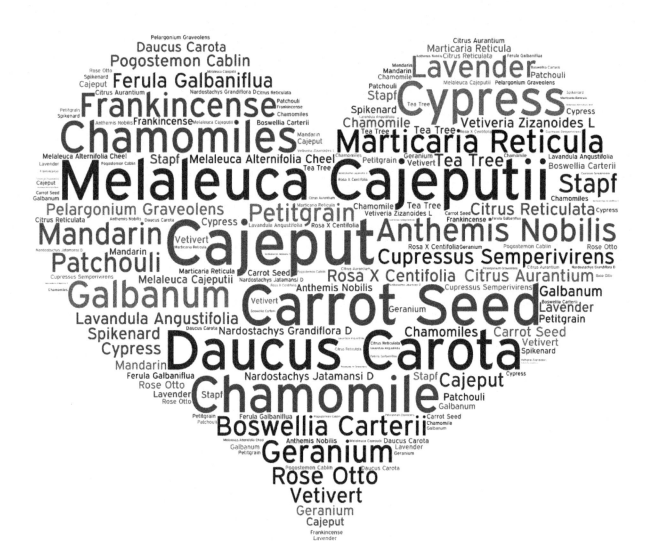

Cajeput (Melaleuca cajeputii)

Carrot Seed (Daucus carota)

Chamomile(s) (Marticaria reticula, Anthemis nobilis)

Cypress (Cupressus semperivirens)

Frankincense (Boswellia carterii)

Galbanum (Ferula galbaniflua)

Geranium (Pelargonium graveolens)

Lavender (Lavandula angustifolia)

Mandarin (Citrus reticulata)

Patchouli (Pogostemon cablin)

Petitgrain (Citrus aurantium)

Rose Otto (Rosa x centifolia)

Spikenard (Nardostachys jatamansi D.C.Nardostachys grandiflora D.C.)

Tea Tree (Melaleuca alternifolia Cheel)

Vetivert (Vetiveria zizanoides L. Stapf.)

Introduction

The stillest point of a seesaw is at its pivoting centre.

I learnt to meditate many years ago. Then, meditation was regarded as a 'fringe' or 'hippy-type' practice, encapsulated and epitomised by media images of the Beatles sat with the Maharishi. Meditation has not changed my destiny or my life's lessons, but it is an invaluable tool, consistently grounding my sense of reality, anchoring my psyche when I feel insecure, calming my racing mind and uncluttering my perspective. I do not meditate every day, but whenever I do the experience is unconditional, unfailing, always 'just there' if I choose to notice, to focus my awareness. Mindfulness is a meditative construct similarly applied as a tool, to the same end; the cup that draws water from the well does not itself quench thirst, but is instrumental in access. Mindfulness is an ancient practice which, although steeped in Buddhist philosophy, currently occupies the foreground of 'vogue' acceptance as a non-religious, cost effective, de-stressing, anti anxiety, anti depressant tool, increasingly embraced by mainstream healthcare as a viable self-help remedy that may be safely applied independently or alongside conventional treatments.

Companions of the meditative process and remedies in their own right too, essential oils play an invaluable complementary role, particularly when utilising their psycho-emotional properties. Essential oils that possess qualities particularly pertinent to meditation and relaxation are described here, with easy-to-follow charts to help you identify their properties and assist and guide your selection.

Meditation

There are various techniques and styles of meditation, however, all meditation appears to share the same universal objective; that is, attainment of a state of inner calm and peace. The key central aim of Mindfulness is simply to 'be', to hone and sustain conscious awareness of 'being' in the present moment:

I shall tell you now and for no extra charge that 'living in the present' seems to be the key component across every scripture, self-help book and religious group I've encountered. To harmonise with life in each moment, not to make happiness contingent on any prospective condition. Not to be tormented by the past but to live in the reality of 'now', all else being mental construct. (Brand 2014 p129-130)

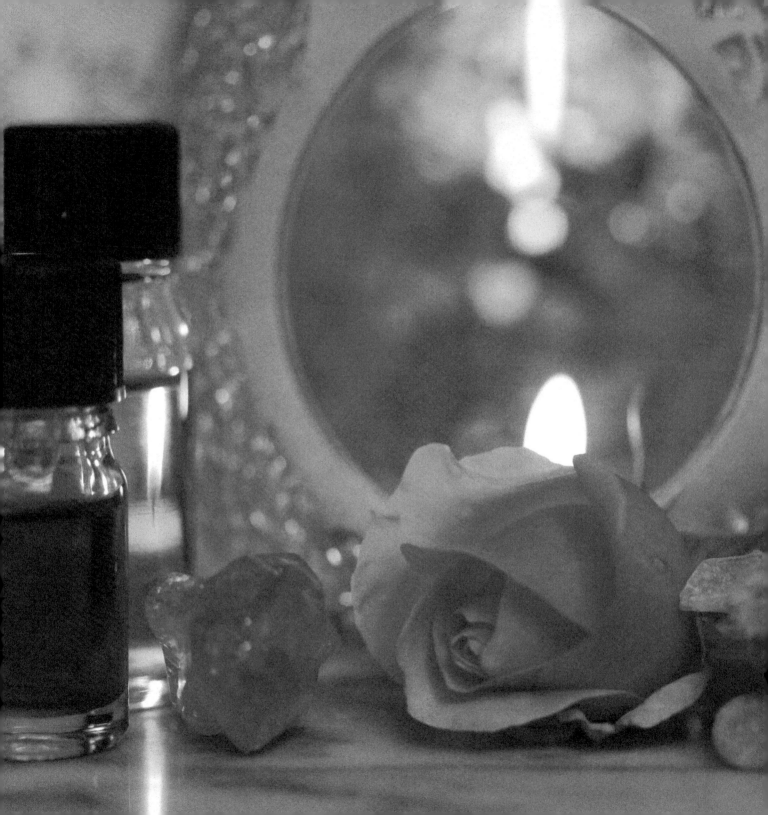

Unconditional consciousness of the present moment naturally disables and dispels thoughts entrenched in the past or future. At the very heart, the epicenter of the 'present moment', past regrets, traumas or disappointments, even joys, future fears, uncertainty, anticipation, expectations, have no place, do not exist. In reality, we actually only ever exist in the present moment. Conscious of 'Being' in the immediacy of 'now' we are more 'awake' to the experience of the world, the environment around us and our immediate inner and outer senses.

Sustaining present moment consciousness ('moment centered consciousness') through meditation appears to bring colour to a sepia picture, as if switching on the light or removing the veiling nets from the window. It allows us to clearly see, experience and sensually observe the richness of what is actually 'here and now'. "En-lightenment". Darkness or shadow cannot exist where there is light. Darkness is the absence of light not the opposite and so is dispelled by light; objects blocking light create a shadow and once they are removed, the shadow no longer exists.

Ruminating thoughts, memories of the past, concerns for the future, worry about an unpaid bill may insidiously move into the foreground of awareness, taking centre stage to fill the frame of consciousness and create shadows. Meditation enables the perceiver to re-evaluate their 'picture', allowing their awareness to encompass the whole scene unimpeded, not just the objects that appear the 'loudest'.

Some argue, however, that concerted focus on the moment may also draw unwelcome attention to or intensify those thoughts or feelings occupying the immediate frame of awareness; as if honing attention appears to consent to their place at centre stage so they seem even more pronounced. It is true, and I speak from personal experience, that for this reason there are times when meditation is not desirable. In such circumstances where unpleasant thoughts, memories, emotional feelings or pain are extremely 'loud' or over-focused, I find deliberate distraction through some other positive activity (physical action or mental concentration) which absorbs my attention provides a more appropriate temporary tool (exercise, walking, painting, reading, watching an enthralling play or film, enjoying the company of good friends, setting a positive itinerary to follow).

Purposefully drawing attention away from the intensity thus allows me to step aside for a moment. My perspective then is able to naturally dissipate more appropriately into context, to calm the exaggerated loudness or brightness. Of course, sometimes the object filling my awareness is there because it does need my attention (hunger, thirst, pain, even the unpaid bill require expedient action). Also, it is possible that distraction can insidiously become, or can be deliberately applied to be, avoidant or denying, a cloak that shrouds from the pain, the fear or whatever the issue is. Such distraction may appear to shield us from the pain and hurt that we believe and fear acknowledgement may expose us to. Sometimes a person requires support, assistance or professional help too. In such circumstances meditation can be used as a complementary tool, when and if we are ready to accept the onus of control. Meditation is a proactive, conscious choice, a gentle process the perceiver may apply:

> *The emphasis on present moment awareness recognizes that this moment is the only moment in which we can act: past moments are only memories that we cannot change directly and future moments are only ideas. But with a realistic appraisal of thoughts, emotions and bodily sensations as they are perceived in the present moment we can move from a passive reactive mode of behavior to one that is infused with initiative and choice. (Burch 2010)*

Russell Brand, above, refers to his experience of Transcendental Meditation (TM). I learned to meditate applying Prem Rawats' (Elan Vital) methods of meditation. Mindfulness is another form of meditation, among many others, which, having demonstrated some success in alleviating the experience of depression, anxiety and post traumatic stress disorder, stress and stress related conditions, is increasingly accepted as a viable self-help remedy. It has been included also in management of chronic pain. Meditation is a voluntary process, which is indeed safe and cost effective but which, more significantly, offers a tool that potentially supports the individual to maintain their personal locus of control, without the unwelcome side effects often associated with taking antidepressant or sedative drugs (although these do, in some instances, play an important role as temporary support). Where drug medication is unavoidably necessary, the concurrent practice of meditation, in some circumstances, has been shown to reduce the quantity required and reduce duration of their prescription.

The Complementary role of Essential oils

Essential oils have accompanied us like guardians and companions on our ever-evolving journey through time and life: applied in the form of fumigants, incense, cleansers, antiseptics, antibiotics, anti-bactericides, preservatives, as well as psychosomatic, hedonistic perfumes, which have not only been worn to adorn, but also to protect, to symbolize intention and to punctuate and accentuate rite and ritual.

Modern scientific investigation, equipment and methodology have enabled greater insight into the practical mechanism, properties, components and chemistry of organic and inorganic matter, providing better understanding of the world around us. It has also taught us much about the physical body and its healthy function, as well as viruses, bacteria, disease and the significant role diet and lifestyle play in supporting and maintaining wellness. As holistic health and wellbeing resurges into the foreground, so too the mind-body-spirit connection is recognized and acknowledged as a significant feature of wellness.

Essential oils continue to be used, as they have throughout history, for their protective, restorative, rehabilitative, hedonistic qualities, seamlessly providing physiological and psycho-emotional-spiritual support and apparently bridging the pragmatic, nature-al and ethereal dynamics of life and existence. In this respect, rather than separating one view from another (reductionism and vitalism), science may contribute, dispelling misguided myth and misbelief, providing insight into the amazing capacity of the body and confirming the complementary relationship and role that plants, energetic medicines and remedies play in assisting maintenance of health and homeostatic balance – the best of both worlds. Indeed, applied as medicine, aesthetically as beautifying ingredients and as spiritual aids, the unifying quality of essential oils provides a link between man, nature and psycho-spiritual realms.

Numerous references are made within historical medicinal texts, treatises and scriptures demonstrating this dynamic role (see, for example, Essential Oils in Therapeutic Context: Historical Background):

Then the Lord said to Moses, "Take fragrant spices - gum resin, onycha and galbanum - and pure frankincense, all in equal amounts, and make a fragrant blend of incense, the work of the perfumer". (Exodus 30:34)

Perfume and incense bring joy to the heart (Proverbs 27:9).

Try and penetrate with our limited means the secrets of nature and you will find that, behind all discernible concatenations, there remains something subtle, intangible and inexplicable. Veneration for the force beyond anything that we can comprehend is my religion. To that extent I am, in point of fact, religious. (Einstein 1927)

Evidenced through their historic and continued use in religious, cultural and spiritual practices, essential oils significantly provide qualities potentially supportive in the context of prayer, intentional focus and meditation. For example, their cephalic, psycho-emotional influence on the limbic system (mood, emotion, calming, sedating, uplifting) and their ability to anchor the recipient into their moment experience through the experiential immediacy of odour awareness, especially when they are deliberately directly inhaled (drops on a tissue, for example) and/or infused into the surrounding environment. Indeed, odour detection forms an ancient, intrinsic facet of human (and animal) survival mechanisms and is powerfully associated with memory. Thus, essential oils can be applied to reinforce memory and to recall events, thoughts and feelings experienced during original odour detection, as well as immediately instilling or procuring attributed psycho-emotional qualities. For example, an essential oil or blend of essential oils

15

diffused and detected during meditation may be deliberately inhaled after the event to trigger recollection of the experience of 'being in' meditation, thus potentially recapturing the sense of stillness and calmness felt 'there and then' in the 'here and now'.

This can act as a reminder to continue to meditate, to maintain conscious awareness of the present moment and to experience feelings of calm and peace 'here and now'. This facet, along with their other significant psycho-emotional qualities, renders essential oils valuable complementary tools, particularly when applied with techniques such as counselling, psychotherapy and cognitive behavioural therapy (CBT), as well as meditation and relaxation techniques. Certain essential oils, frankincense and patchouli for example, regulate breathing, instilling a sense of peace and tranquility and consequently aid in quieting an anxious, 'racing' mind. Other essential oils, such as rose and mandarin, are gently stimulating and uplifting. Yet others, amongst them lavender and geranium, possess both calming and stimulating qualities and are emotionally balancing.

What is Mindfulness?

Mindfulness, an aspect of 'insight meditation', evolved from Buddhism and was introduced into the West during the 1970s. Although steeped in Buddhist philosophy, the simplicity of its processes and practice enables its presentation in non-religious, independent contexts as an aid to focused attention on the 'here and now'; conscious, present-centred awareness amidst the rhythm of daily life.

> So, how much faith do you need? Do you need to convert to Buddhism? Do you need to abandon the tradition in which you were raised or the ideals to which you have deep commitment? Do you need to set aside anything that your intellect or understanding of the world tells you? Absolutely not. You can retain your current frame of reference and accept only what you are prepared to accept, a piece at a time, and only what you in fact find helpful. Yet you do need some faith. You need the same kind of faith that you need to read a good novel or conduct a scientific experiment. You need "a willing suspension of disbelief... faith, which at heart is nothing more than the willingness to accept provisionally something without yet having proved or verified it for oneself". (Gunarantana 2009 p 1,2)

Mindful Awareness (vipassana) is a state of consciously being aware, 'paying attention' to, maintaining concentration on and consciousness of the 'here and now', 'being' in the present moment; noticing what is happening internally and externally without pre-judgement, condition or expectation, but with gentle acceptance, unconditional intentionality and equanimity (calmness of temper, composure).

> Mindfulness is a way of being aware – mindful awareness is receptive not exclusive. Sensations, thoughts or feelings are simply experienced for what they are. To be mindfully aware means, strangely, there can be no 'mind'. Even if thoughts are chattering away, they receive no more attention than anything else that has arisen. As people's ordinary, reactive ways of restricting their awareness diminishes, a sense of the suchness of things emerges. (Mace 2007 p 1)

Meditation per se is an experiential process that apparently provides a bridge between the finite and infinite (or the deepest sense of inner 'being'). In this sense the meditator may evolve through various phases, or layers, of consciousness, from physical finite awareness to states of deep, wordless inner awareness, enlightening realisation and

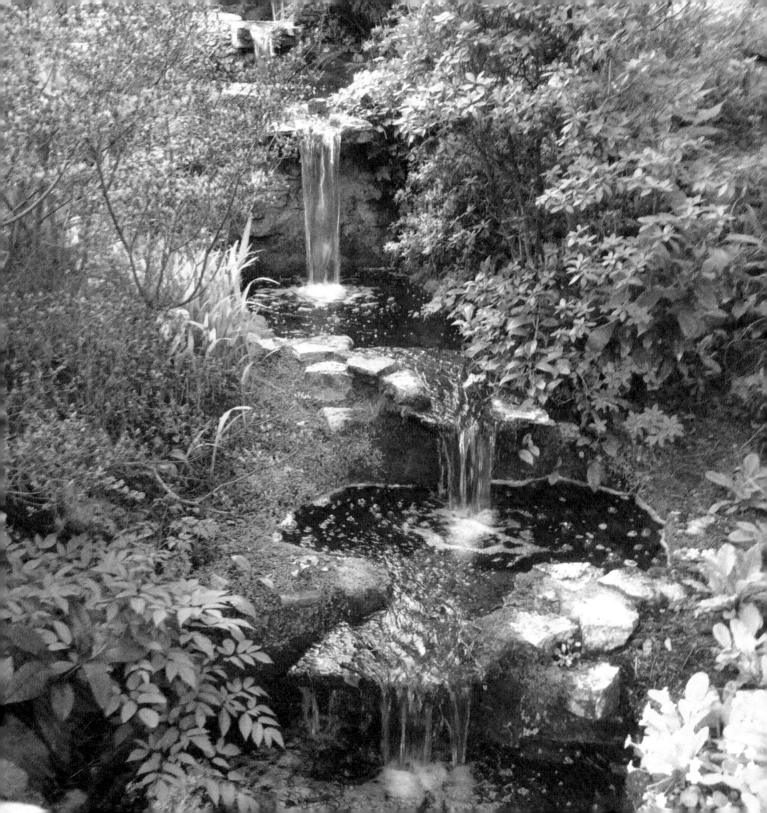

deep understanding… "wordless, not conveyed or perceived as idea or thought in our ordinary meaning of those words but as immediate, direct, shapeless and formless realisation in and by holistic consciousness... later [given] shape and form as inspired idea and word." (Mehta 1989 p 36).

The techniques of mindful attention or intentionality take the perceiver to the well but the techniques are not the water; the water (experience) drawn from the well and contained within the cup (mindful attention) offers a taste, an insight, of the ocean; or put differently, the 'cup' represents our finite language and physical experience and can only contain, or process through language and feeling, a limited amount of 'water' from the well – an elephant does not fit into a matchbox. Put differently again, the body (physical and spiritual) might be seen as the well, techniques of meditation, or concentrated focus, the cup that enables the perceiver to draw from the inner depths of the well; awareness of innate and infinite 'spirit' within (not outside, above or beyond, but inside and available).

Kabat Zinn (2004 p 1) observes the 'miracle of the five senses as tools which ground and anchor and enable access to full awareness and appreciation of the moment experience, "seeing that which is here to be seen, hearing that which is here to be heard, etc. - the five senses plus what the Buddha included as the sixth and most important and unifying sense, which is the capacity of the mind itself for nonconceptual knowing." Being aware in the moment and holding that awareness by anchoring to the immediacy of what is felt, sensed and observed, internally and externally, brings the perceiver to the gateway of consciousness awareness, of simply 'being'. Practicing mindful awareness enables a focusing of attention on the 'here and now'. Simply 'being' within the moment experience potentially instils a sense of peace, completeness and acceptance (among other qualities) – a wordless sense of the fullness of existence.

Research evidence examining brain images during the process of meditation demonstrates significant consequential neural response, indicating that regular meditation practice aids in positive re-structure of negative self narrative, thoughts, attitudes and behaviours in a way that enhances self-compassion, positive self-image and reduced feelings of anxiety, depression and ruminating thoughts. Essential oils stimulate and influence similar neural pathways and areas within the brain, thus sharing some affinity with the practice of meditation, particularly when considering their ability to sedate, calm, ground and uplift the recipient. However, largely due to a lack of funding, there is limited or no similar brain-imaging research evidence available to verify (or disprove) this affinity to date.

Mindful Awareness is a way of being, a moment-to-moment experience best appreciated through regular, daily attention, compassionate self discipline and tenacity; the impact more fully appreciated when practice is frequent and regular, for example 'little and often' rather than once a week or 'every so often'. Mindful Awareness and Meditation precedes deeper meditative states, thus the consequence of mindfulness may extend beyond merely providing a coping strategy or relaxation technique to apply during stressful periods of life. Crisis often acts as a catalyst for change – for example, introduced as a coping tool, the experiential process of Mindful Awareness and Meditation may consequently lead to enlightened discovery of a sense, an awareness of 'presence' and 'being' previously never considered, or overlooked, as Shapiro et al (2002 p 634) acknowledge:

> "formal meditation seeps into daily life, bringing greater non-judgemental consciousness to everything that one does, feels and experiences."

To reiterate, there are two identifiable modes of Mindfulness: **Awareness Practice** and **Meditation**.

Awareness Practice

Mindful Practice, or **Intentional Awareness (vipassana)**, focuses on being awake to what is happening in the immediacy of 'here and now', noticing what is being felt, observed or experienced in any given moment, internally and externally. This is achieved by employing the mind to 'check' focused attention:

> Clear comprehension means remaining fully awake and conscious in the midst of any activity, everything your body is doing and everything you are perceiving. It is a turned-within monitoring of everything going on in the mind and body. Clear comprehension requires 'bare attention' ("bare" in the sense of stripped down or nothing added over the top) to assure that you are mindful of the right things and mindful in the right way. It is a quality control factor that monitors what is being noticed and how the noticing is taking place. (Gunaratana 2009 p17).

So, to elaborate, here and now I am sitting at my table with my hands poised on the keyboard of my lap top. I feel the breeze entering the barge through the open window brushing against my face as I concentrate on typing these words. I hear a distant duck quacking, the sound of the wind blowing against the half open window shutter, rustling the leaves in the trees outside, the cars in the distance humming. I notice the fading light around me as the sun sets outside, the birds twittering, that my neck and shoulders are aching from holding the same position for too long. I notice the bitter, pungent taste in my mouth of the coffee I drank a moment ago, its flavour still on my breath. I feel the pressure of the chair against my bottom, my feet on the soft rug lying across the solid wooden floor.

As I focus on these immediate sensations (all be it in 'scattered' observation), I am aware that I feel peaceful. I notice I am conscious of my breathing and feel the softness and

20

warmth of the air as it passes through my nose into my throat, warmly filling my lungs, then rising and exiting down my nose. In this moment my sense of peace is comforting and fulfilling. Using the immediacy of this sensual check I am brought to the gate of conscious awareness and in this state of conscious awareness I find myself in peace. I can do this as an exercise, following a less 'scattered', prescribed routine of 'noticing', perhaps as a body scan. Or, I can find a starting point and then allow my experience to emerge as I focus attention on a selected object or point within my vision, holding the object in steady view while allowing my consciousness, my vision, to remain open to the whole peripheral territory, noticing at the same time what I feel inside, in my body, my rambling thoughts, my physical sensations; no resistance, but observation, acknowledgment, acceptance. I can practice this focused attention at phases during the day, to anchor myself to the moment, to hone my awareness to the present, as I find myself distracted and drawn into events around me; noticing as I eat my food, wash the dishes, walk to the car, sit in discourse with my students; "bare attention", unconditional and non-judgemental.

Focus on present-awareness, on being in the moment, is also applied as a tool in Gestalt Therapy, Cognitive Behavioural Therapy and Counselling. Fromm (1998 p 39, 95), for example, pertinently observes:

> ...it is important to see the patient [client] as the hero of a drama and not to see him [or her] as a summation of complexes. And, actually, every human being is the hero of a drama... seeing, feeling, sensing, becoming aware enables mobilisation of energy to do something about it... energy can become focused, deliberately directed, effective.

This perspective holds true for and encapsulates the essence of most 'helping professions', particularly Integrative Therapies such as Acupuncture, Essential Oil Therapy, Bowen, Yoga, Counselling and Cognitive Behavioural Therapy (CBT), as well as Mindful Awareness and Practice. Significantly Fromm (1998 – 89) acknowledges:

> Mindfulness means awareness. I am fully aware at every moment of my body, including my posture, anything that goes on in my body, and I am fully aware of my thoughts, of what I think; I am fully concentrated.

Mindful Awareness Practice is incorporated intentionally to anchor a client (or individual) into their present moment experience, especially pertinent when working with various conditions, for example, anxiety and depression and post traumatic stress disorder (PTSD), where a grounded sense of the present, a point to start at and return to in cyclical exploratory journeying and closure, is significant.

Rogers (1980) reiterates this, relating to the significance of the counsellor being present and aware in a conscious state of acceptance that is underpinned by the condition of being in congruence, positive regard and empathy, maintaining awareness and attention while they 'walk alongside their client' in the present moment:

> *"...when we provide a psychological climate that permits a person to be... we are tapping into a tendency which permeates all organic life..." (Rogers 1980 p 134).*

Meditation

Deep concentration meditation (shamatha) is the second mode of Mindfulness (although some prefer to refer to 'gentle awareness' rather than 'deep concentration' to accentuate the sense of choice underpinning this practice). As previously mentioned, Mindfulness Awareness practice is a prerequisite. Again, this process requires self-discipline and is rewarded with an enriched, deeper spiritual understanding and/or sense of 'what is'.

There are four specific underpinning elements, or 'foundations', of focus applied to hone this deeper concentration meditation:

- Mindfulness of the body.
- Mindfulness of feelings.
- Mindfulness of consciousness.
- Mindfulness of mental objects.

These four foundational 'pillars' provide the corner stones of the 'Noble Eightfold Path', which encapsulate a formula to guide, discipline, support and direct intentional mindful focus. This formula is broadly divided into three intentional categories:

- Moral conduct.
- Right concentration.
- Right wisdom.

However, just as with 'the elephant and the blind men', (each feeling a different part of the elephant - the trunk, the foot, the ear, the tail - and proclaiming 'an elephant is like a snake or a drum' etc.) there is some variance in the language selected between authors to depict these qualities, demonstrated in the example overleaf:

The Noble Eightfold Path	
Gunaratana (2009 p 33, 34)	Mace (2008 p 9)
1. Right view 2. Right resolve 3. Right speech 4. Right action 5. Right livelihood 6. Right effort 7. Right mindfulness 8. Right concentration	1. Attainment of morality (sita) 2. Concentration (samadhi) 3. Wisdom (panna) The factors that make for concentration are: 1 Right effort 2 Right awareness (Mindfulness is an essential ingredient of 'right awareness') 3 Right concentration 4 Right understanding 5 Right thought Three essential interdependent characteristics are: 1. Unsatisfactoriness (suffering) (dukka) 2. Transience (anicca) 3. Absence of self (annatta)
Mindfulness Qualities	
Synder & Lopez, 2007)	(Shapiro et al, 2002)
Acceptance Empathy Generosity Gentleness Gratitude Letting go	Loving kindness Non-judging Non-striving Openness Patience Trust

In spite of variance in the descriptive language selected, the overarching core themes emanating from the above appear to provide a general formula for **correct behaviour** and **attitude (conduct)**, **right concentration** and **right mindfulness (wisdom)**. The outcome of this, as Gunaratana (2009) expresses, is 'bright wakefulness', or, as Shapiro et al (2002 p 634) suggest "the intention behind meditation is to "wake up" from this suboptimal state ["normality" or "developmental arrest" (Walsh 1993)] of consciousness, to wake up to our true nature."

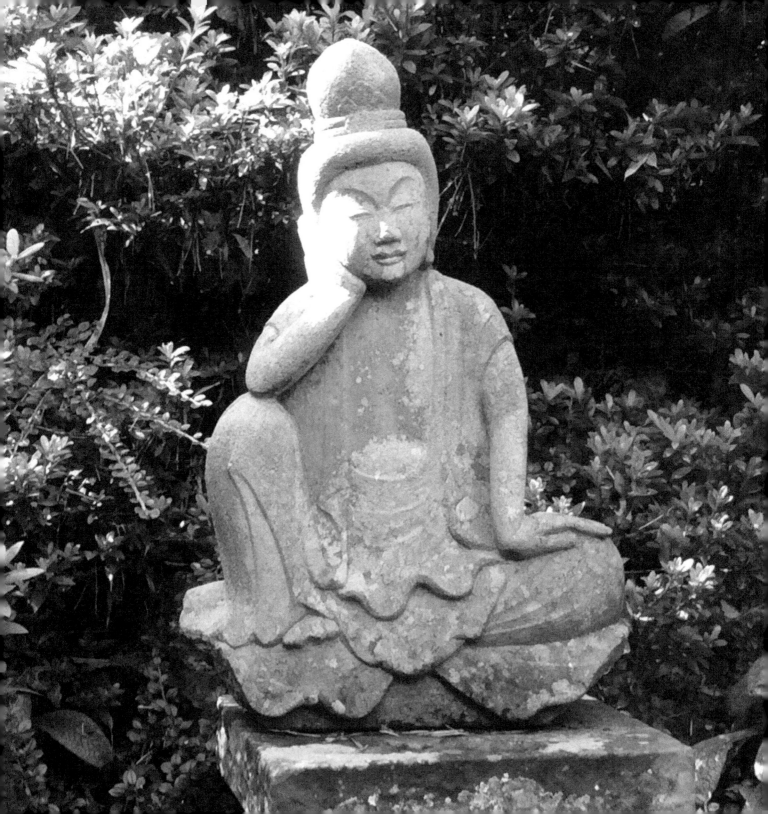

Mindfulness Meditation

Rinpoche (2010) recommends meditating for ten to twenty minutes twice a day in a place that is not too noisy or distracting, sitting cross legged or on a chair with feet touching the ground, holding or supporting a straight back, then gazing a few inches in front of the face, eyes lowered, focusing on an object and/or the breath. Unlike Mindful Awareness Practice, peripheral vision is not embraced beyond the object of gazing. Holding the gaze, the mind is gently brought back from wandering to the object of focus and/or concentration of the breath, which is gentle and unforced. The intention is to achieve 'peace of mind', 'compassionate awareness' and to allow this condition of awareness to permeate the consciousness of 'being'.

Mindful Awareness Practice (intentional awareness), even though steeped in Buddhist philosophy, is not intended to be religious (although there is apparently, probably inevitably, a connotative element of 'spirituality'). Practice requires consistency but not obsession, rite or ritual (although sometimes rite and ritual act as reminders that may superficially assist discipline, it is important to remember that there is a difference between discipline and obsession). Advocates of this process suggest that Mindfulness Practice and Meditation may coexist with other beliefs or may be used and practiced independent of any belief.

Mindfulness Practice is a practical, simple process which merely supports concentration on the 'here and now' and the experience of simply 'being'. It is true, though, that the 'temporary suspension of disbelief' does appear to require a certain amount of faith, held at least long enough to allow the consequential experience of mindfulness practice to manifest, especially as this is not always immediately obvious; only through continual gentle practice do the consequential effects begin to emerge into the foreground of conscious awareness, "seeping into daily life, bringing greater non-judgemental consciousness to everything that one does, feels and experiences." (Shapiro et al 2002 p 634).

The subtle simplicity of Mindfulness, however, does raise academic debate, especially as even among the various Buddhist traditions there is variance in descriptive terms (for example, concentration versus gentle awareness). Chamber et al (2009 p 562) question whether "mindfulness represents a distinct construct or a quality of consciousness that spans and incorporates other states", identifying two potential dimensions to mindfulness practice: pre-thought present moment experience and secondary processing, where thought-awareness (or cognitive interpretation) identifies conditions such as acceptance and non-judgment, thus deviating from the condition of complete pre-thought, present-centred, non-judgemental awareness.

This disparity equally lends itself to the authors, the deliverers (teachers or guides) and receivers (students, clients or readers) interpretational perspective (spiritual, religious and personal values). Evaluative description, for example, is conveyed through the lens (and language) of the experiencer's own relationship with the process (again, the elephant and the blind men). This slant may potentially influence expression and formulation of prescribed practical processes, description and portrayal of information - somehow the 'just being' element becomes shrouded or obscured, even lost (perhaps like when trying to grasp a slippery piece of soap) in trying to emotionally and cognitively understand, justify and describe the process, to attempt to tangibly make 'sense' of its practice and experience. To avoid this ambiguity and confusion, Gunaratana (2009) recommends it is better to say what mindfulness does rather than trying to explain what it is. For example, the practice of mindfulness, as with any meditation technique, initially involves tangible and practical processes, such as the act of focusing on an object, and the outcome of practicing meditation is observable, comparable and measurable, for example, improved concentration, calmness and equanimity.

What mindfulness 'does'

Shapiro et al (2002 p 634) suggest that Buddhist theory and Mindfulness appear to complement and share some affinity with psychology, especially the quality of encouraging positive personal 'self' awareness, and that as such "meditation provides road maps to reach optimal openness, awareness and insight". For example, Mace (2008), reporting on a study conducted by Kutz et al (1985) of twenty patients using mindfulness alongside psychotherapy, observed an overall reduction in negativity and anxiety (although they also observed that hostility, relationships, family and sexual adjustment and emotional inhibition generally appeared unaffected). Significantly, Kutz et al noted some change through the course of meditation, which involved a capacity to access feelings and memories that had not been visited for years, improvements in insight and the capacity to continue to use therapy productively, suggesting these traits do indicate the viable, cost-effective potential of integrating mindfulness practice alongside other therapeutic approaches.

Goldin et al (2009), in a study examining the effects of mindfulness-based stress reduction (MBSR) on the brain behaviour mechanism of self-referential processing in fourteen patients with social anxiety disorder, observed increased self esteem and

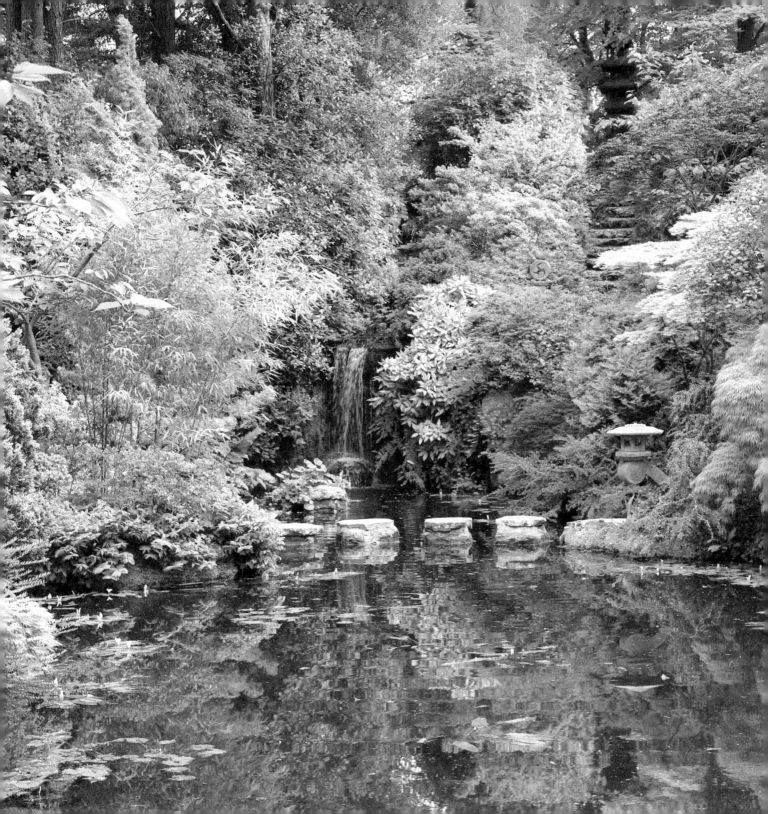

decreased anxiety, increased positive and decreased negative self-endorsement, increased activity in areas of the brain related to attention regulation and reduced activity in brain systems implicated in conceptual-linguistic self-view. They suggest the practice of MBSR techniques may have a positive influence on maladjusted or distorted social self-view, potentially related to changes in the way people view themselves and their ability to maintain attention. This is explained as a result of positively rephrasing internal dialogue and consciously breaking the habit of internal negative narrative. Regularly engaging in Mindfulness practice actually altered neural pathways and areas of activity within the brain, ultimately reprogramming self-defeating tendencies and dialogue that reinforced negative behaviour, thus providing capacity for and enabling positive self-perspective.

Mackenzie et al (2006) found that nurses and nurses aides, recruited from long-term complex continuing care units in a large geriatric teaching hospital in America, and engaged in a programme of Mindfulness practice, experienced significant improvements in burnout symptoms, relaxation and life satisfaction compared to a control waiting-list group. Consequently, their recommendation was that Mindfulness practice offered a promising method of managing stress amongst staff. Similarly, Shapiro et al (2005), in a study involving healthcare professionals (nurses, social workers, physiotherapists and psychologists) who participated in a MBSR programme, reported decrease in perceived stress and greater self-compassion when compared with controls ('compassion' is encapsulated in the list of Mindful Qualities).

Reported psychological distress, dissatisfaction with life and job burnout were also decreased, although the differences between the experimental and the control groups were not significant in this respect. However, participants did indicate that the MBSR programme had a substantially positive impact on their lives. The authors did report a significantly higher than average (20%) dropout rate at 44% - dropout participants attributed their departure from the programme to difficulty in managing their workload as well as being involved in the study, especially in view of the limited time available to them!

Wang et al (2010) found that the frontal regions, anterior cingulate cortex, limbic system and parietal lobes within the brain (see Absorption, Characteristics and Application: Essential Oil Gems) were affected during meditative states, noting strong correlations between depth of meditation and neural activity in the left inferior forebrain relating to the subjective experience of the meditators. Holzel et al (2010), in a study examining the neural effect of a MBSR programme on sixteen healthy, meditation-naive participants, observed increases in gray matter concentration within the left hippocampus. Whole brain analysis identified increases in the posterior cingulate cortex, the temporo-parietal junction and the cerebellum in the MBSR group compared with the controls; thus indicating changes in brain regions involved in learning and memory process, emotion regulation, self-referential processing and perspective taking.

Goldin et al (2009) (mentioned previously), supporting this result, identified positive correlation between brain activity in the prefrontal region of the brain from neuro-images taken of patients with Social Anxiety Disorder pre and during mindfulness appraisal; MBSR resulted in moderate reduction of symptoms of social anxiety, depression, ruminating thoughts, states of anxiety and increased self esteem.

Such results confirm the potential to positively change or re-programme neural mechanisms through Mindfulness practice. Engaging in regular practice of meditation appears to have a calming effect, which may permeate beyond the duration and state of being in meditation. Negative self-defeating narrative and thought patterns, attitude, perception and behaviour may be reversed or improved through being suspended in the experience of 'being' in a positive, unthreatened state during meditation, and through deliberate positive internal affirmation; retraining or retuning neural pathways. This positive sense of being whole and complete irrespective of the condition (anxiety, depression, ruminating thoughts, physical pain), being consciously calm and self-approving through employing the mindful qualities of kindness and compassion, enables a person to identify their true locus of control. Thus the present-centered quality of Mindfulness does appear effective in alleviating anxiety and supporting improved self-image and perception; anchoring the perceiver to their present-moment experience paradoxically also appears to instigate a journey of renewed self-discovery.

Personal Reflection

Having practiced meditation for more than forty years (although duration or length of time in the context of meditation is not relevant as it is always a 'moment' experience), I do recognise many of the elements described in the literature regarding the experience of Mindful Awareness Practice and Meditation. The meditation I was taught focuses on techniques that hone attention inwardly and, like Mindfulness, is not attached to a specific religion. Similarly, consciousness of 'being in the moment' is a significant feature, as well as the ability to surrender, let go and allow consciousness of the experience of meditating to permeate awareness. This meditation is also very simple. The only condition is the regular practice of the meditation techniques; there is no doctrine. As with Mindfulness, it is an experiential process, which only in proactively engaging yields the consequential appreciation and feeling of connectedness and peace:

> *"Peace needs to be in everyone's life. It is not the world that needs peace, it is people. When people in the world are at peace within, the world will be at peace. The peace that we are looking for is within. It is in the heart, waiting to be felt..."*
> *(Prem Rawat 2011).*

Because the practice of these techniques is so familiar, I find myself naturally slipping into the breathing technique I was taught when I practice Mindful Awareness. Indeed, breath focus features in all meditative processes and techniques of relaxation. However, in some instances, breath focus is undesirable (for example, during anxiety and panic attacks or in Obsessive Compulsive Disorder), as focused attention on breathing can exacerbate a tendency for over-breathing, panic or an obsessive need to control, or may remind a person of previous experiences of being in such states and so trigger a similar response (mental distraction from being over focused is best employed in these circumstances). Concentration on meditation is not forced or rigid, but gentle, achieved through compassionate awareness, rather than military-like prescription, discipline, obsession and regime.

I find the practice of Mindful Awareness useful in preparing myself prior to and ending formal meditation. Although I practice Mindful Awareness intermittently during the day, this is automatically, seamlessly accompanied by my conscious awareness of the meditation breathing technique I have practiced for years; one seems to enhance the other. I am not always in a state of Mindful Awareness or meditation, but I do have a choice and, in returning my attention to either, I am aware that whatever I am concentrating on, my experience of being is always constantly, conditionlessly there. I find the techniques of Mindful Awareness a practical, tangible construct; deliberately noticing, paying attention to internal and external sensations and experience does provide a road map (Shapiro et al 2002), a point of reference to direct my awareness and dialogue in aiding my attention toward my own moment focus, reminding me to remain in a state of present centred consciousness.

I also notice that if I diffuse an essential oil or blend of essential oils during the formal process of meditation, I am able to recall the experience of calmness felt if I smell this odour later in the day as I attend to other things. This in turn inspires or reminds me to remain aware of 'being' in the moment, to hold this sense of calmness and awareness of 'there and then' renewed in the 'here and now'. Remaining conscious of 'being' in the present moment I am at the 'gateway', the bridge, between finite and infinite awareness; holding, with compassion, this awareness of 'being here and now' dissolves the veil of separation.

Traditionally, most prescribed Mindfulness Stress Reduction Programmes run in eight-week blocks and generally consist of two-hour sessions once a week and daily one hour independent meditation practice; thus, having established a pattern or habit of Mindful Awareness and Meditation, the attendee is equipped to continue independently. Rinpoche (2010), as previously mentioned, recommends meditating twice a day (morning and evening), in ten to twenty minute sessions (with compassionate acceptance if this routine is broken through other more immediate needs and demands – i.e. being self disciplined rather than obsessional), initially focusing on one of the following:

Initial pre-meditation Mindfulness focus

Body Scan   Progressively moving attention from the toes to the head (or head to toes), observing any sensations in the different regions of the body

Yoga   Stretches and postures designed to enhance greater awareness of and to balance and strengthen the musculoskeletal system

Mindful Practice   Focusing on an object and the breath and the peripheral environment / noticing what is happening in the present moment (seeing / hearing / sensing / tasting / feeling / touching / walking / sitting / preparing food / getting dressed etc.)

Sitting in Meditation   Holding gentle focus on an object. Being aware of body sensations, thoughts and emotions while continually returning the focus of attention to the breath

In mindfulness, or shamatha, meditation, we are trying to achieve a mind that is stable and calm. What we begin to discover is that this calmness or harmony is a natural aspect of the mind. Through mindfulness practice we are just developing and strengthening it and eventually we are able to remain peacefully in our mind without struggling. Our mind naturally feels content.

(Rinpoche 2010)

Essential oils can be used prior to meditation as part of your preparation process (perhaps in a bath, self-massage oil blend, or simply environmentally vapourised in a diffuser). They can be used during meditation to aid concentration, focus, alertness, 'wakefulness', and to calm racing thoughts and ease restlessness (perhaps applied as a personal perfume or, again, diffused into the atmosphere). Post meditation, essential oils can be used as a memory cue, a gentle reminder to return attention to the 'here and now' or for their physiological and psycho-emotional uplifting, grounding and balancing qualities. Your selection of essential oils will be personal and pertinent to you and what you require or need; there is not a 'perfect blend' in this context but for the one that works best for you at any given moment in time. Your own 'nose' will help you discover the 'alchemist within'; your instinct and intuition is a good starting point.

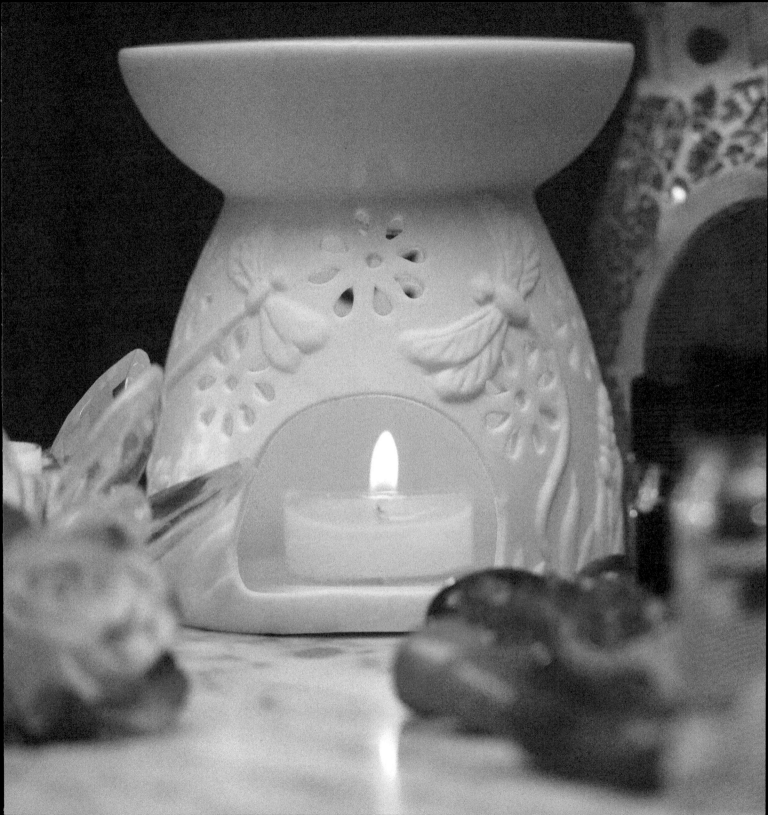

Essential oils – meditation companions

Essential Oil 'Gems' represent the least hazardous oils and, collectively, complement each other's qualities well. They possess invaluable characteristics pertinent to supporting meditation, concentration, relaxation and clarity. These essential oils feature among those most frequently selected by my clients to aid their relaxation and their ability to de-stress and to alleviate related symptoms such as insomnia, anxiety and depression, among others.

Indeed, Essential Oil 'Gems' feature among those that appear in the historical canons, treatises, medicinal and philosophical texts of ancient civilisations (from the Ancient Chinese and Egyptians to Middle Age herbalists, alchemists and perfumers), passed on and recorded by shamans, priests, healers and early doctors across time and continents. Numerous references to essential oils, scented flowers, herbs and spices are made within various scriptures including, among others, the Rig and Artharva Veda, the Quaran, the Bhagavad-Gita and the Bible. The Bible, for example, mentions several historic essences used to heal, cleanse, protect and to symbolize prayer and religious ritual. These essences, balsams and incense were mainly extracted from crushed or infused roots, bark, twigs and leaves, gums and resins exuding from plants and trees.

Essential oils (resins, gums, essences and incense) referred to in the Bible include:

Balm of Gilead (*Pistacia lentiscus*) Benzoin Styrax (*Styrax benzoin*) Calamus (*Acorus calamus*) Cassia (*Cinnamomum cassia*)	Cedarwood (*Cedrus atlantica*) Cinnamon (*Cinnamomum zeylanicum*) Frankincense (Olibanum) (*Boswelia carterii*) Galbanum (*Ferula galbaniflua*)	Labdanum (Cistus) (rock rose, onycha) (*Cistus ladaniferus*) Myrrh (ancient mimosa?) (*Commiphora myrrh*) Sandalwood (possible cross reference with aloewood, oud, oodh, agar) (*Santalum album*) Spikenard (nard) (*Nardostotachys jatamansi*)

References		
Exodus 30:22-25, 30:34 Esther 2:12 Isaiah 55:13, 60:6 Jeremiah 6:20, 8:22 John 19:39 Leviticus 2:1, 2:16, 6:16, 14:4, 14:6, 14:49, 14:51, 14:52, 24:7	Luke 1:10 Malachi 1:11 Mark 14:3 Matthew 2:11 Nehemiah 8:15 Numbers 16:46-48, 19:6, 24:6	Philippians 4:18 Proverbs 7:17, 27:9 Psalm 45:8, 51:7, 141:2 Revelations 5:8, 8:3 Solomon 1:3, 1:12, 3:6, 4:6, 4:11- 14, 4: 13-15, 4:40

Continuing Lord Krishna states that He enters into every particle of earth with His energy, prevailing over all the Earth with His prowess and supports all moving and non-moving jivas or embodied beings. He, Himself, is the luminosity of moonlight which nourishes all herbs and crops such as rice, fruits and grains. (Rudra Vaisnava Sampradaya, Sridhara Swami Commentary: Srimad Bhagavad-Gita 15:13)

Your plants are an orchard of pomegranates with choice fruits, with henna and nard, nard and saffron, calamus and cinnamon, with every kind of incense tree, with myrrh and aloes and all the finest spices. You are a garden fountain, a well of flowing water streaming down from Lebanon.(Songs of Solomon 4: 13-15)

Breath was considered the portal of consciousness, the connection between the world and the Divine, the connection between the soul and the manifest material universe, the bridge between the world and the spirit within (consciousness). Breath is vital, it sustains life force. Odour, through the ages, has been employed to stimulate awareness of this connection, of our 'spiritual' self. Incense and resins were burned during rites, rituals, ceremonies, prayer – the smoke symbolising the soul, consciousness, rising toward heaven or the higher self; 'god' awareness. Such rites and rituals were originally performed to remind the observer to remain focused on their breath; to remain consciously connected to awareness of the omniscience of 'god'.

Essential oil molecules, carried within the breath, sweep across the olfactory bulbs, sending neural messages registered within the brain, detected by consciousness, connecting awareness to the nuances of the external and internal world. The immediacy of odour detection, the act of deliberately smelling scent, draws the perceiver's consciousness to their breathing, to the moment.

All Essential Oil Gems potentially support meditation, but especially Cypress, Frankincense, Galbanum , Patchouli, Rose Otto and Spikenard

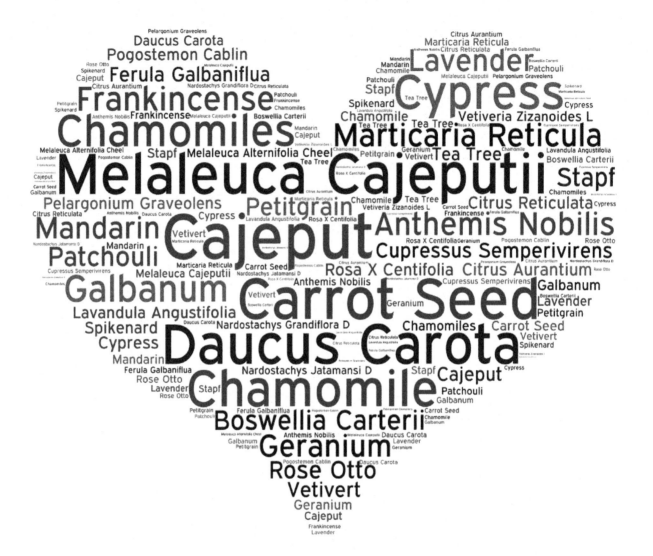

What is an Essential Oil? How do they support meditation?

Essential oils are highly concentrated, volatile, odiferous phytochemical derivatives extracted from various parts of certain plants, trees and shrubs: for example, rhizomes and roots, stems, leaves, flowering heads, seeds, wood (stumps, trunk, heartwood, sawdust), twigs, bark, resin, needles, berries, blossoms, fruit, rind and grass. Not all plants produce essential oils. According to Tisserand and Young (2014), and Lawrence (1995), there are an estimated 350,000 plant species existent throughout the world, of which just 17,500 (5%) are aromatic; 400 of these aromatic species surrender essential oils suitable for commercial use; 50% are specifically cultivated for their essential oil, while others are grown, managed and harvested in the wild. Many essential oils are produced as a by-product of industry (for example, citrus oils such as orange, lemon and lime, produced for the food, manufacturing and perfume industries).

Examples of areas where essential oils are stored within the plant ('Gem' essential oils highlighted).

Bark	Cinnamon
Berries	Juniper
Blossom	Neroli (orange), jasmine, rose, ylang ylang
Flowers	Calendula, **chamomile German & Roman**, clove bud, helichrysum
	Flowering tops
	Hyssop, **lavender**, lemon balm, marjoram, peppermint, rosemary, clary sage, thyme
Fruits	Black pepper, litsea cubeba (May Chang), star anise
Grass (leaves)	Citronella, lemongrass, palmarosa
Leaves	**Cajeput**, cinnamon, eucalyptus, hyssop, **lavender**, lemon balm, myrtle, niaouli, **patchouli**, peppermint, **petitgrain**, rosemary, sage, clary sage, **tea tree**, thyme
Needles	**Cypress**, pine
Resins	**Frankincense**, **galbanum**, myrrh, tolu balsam
Rind	Bergamot, grapefruit, lemon, lime, **mandarin**, orange bitter
Roots, rhizomes	Angelica, ginger, **spikenard**, valerian, **vetivert**
Seeds	Caraway, cardamom, **carrot seed**, coriander, fennel, bitter fennel, nutmeg
Twigs, branches	**Cajeput**, cinnamon, **cypress**, eucalyptus, myrtle, niaouli, **petitgrain**, **tea tree**
Whole plant	(above ground) Bitter fennel, **geranium**, rosemary (poor quality), yarrow
Wood	(stumps, trunk, heartwood, sawdust) Cedarwood, rosewood, sandalwood

How are essential oils absorbed by the body?

There are three ways in which essential oils may enter the body:

Oral ingestion (also including rectal or vaginal absorption via suppositories).

Olfaction (inhalation).

Percutaneous (skin) absorption.

Percutaneous absorption will not be covered in this book, but is covered in depth in 'Essential Oil Gems: Absorption, Characteristics and Application'.

Oral ingestion

Oral ingestion is not recommended unless prescribed and administered by a primary healthcare practitioner who is also a trained and qualified essential oil practitioner; I do not advocate oral ingestion of essential oils in any other circumstance. There are numerous cautionary contributory factors to consider when ingesting essential oils orally. It is likely that when administered orally 95 - 100% of the essential oil ingested will be absorbed into the body's internal system (unlike skin absorption, where the epidermis acts as a semi porous barrier). Essential oils should never be swallowed neat because they can cause severe mucous membrane irritation.

Although essential oils are metabolised and eliminated or excreted from the body quite quickly, there is increased risk of causing renal (kidney) and hepatic (liver) damage and internal irritation to other accessory organs of the digestive system. Some essential oils are oral toxins. There is also increased risk of negative chemical interaction between the constituents of essential oils and other prescribed medication that may be being taken at the same time, which might potentiate or exacerbate their action. For example, sweet birch or wintergreen essential oil should never be administered internally if a person is also taking Warfarin, as these essential oils dangerously increase the anti-coagulant and blood thinning potential of Warfarin.

In other examples, Tisserand and Young (2014) warn of possible incompatibility between oral ingestion of chaste tree, cypress (blue), sandalwood (W. Australian) essential oils and jasmine sambac absolute (Latin names not given), and tricyclic antidepressants, such as imipramine and amitriptyline, or opiates such as codeine, among other CYP2D6 substrates: essential oils can potentiate the action of these drugs (inhalation and topical dermal application of balsam poplar, chamomile blue, sage and yarrow may also potentiate the action of CYP2D6 substrate drugs).

Olfactory Absorption (Inhalation)

Olfaction refers to the nose and the process of the sense of smell. As a method of absorption, olfaction lends itself well to the highly volatile, odiferous nature of essential oils. Olfactory absorption (inhalation) is generally described below and relates most significantly to meditation.

The olfactory pathways into the brain

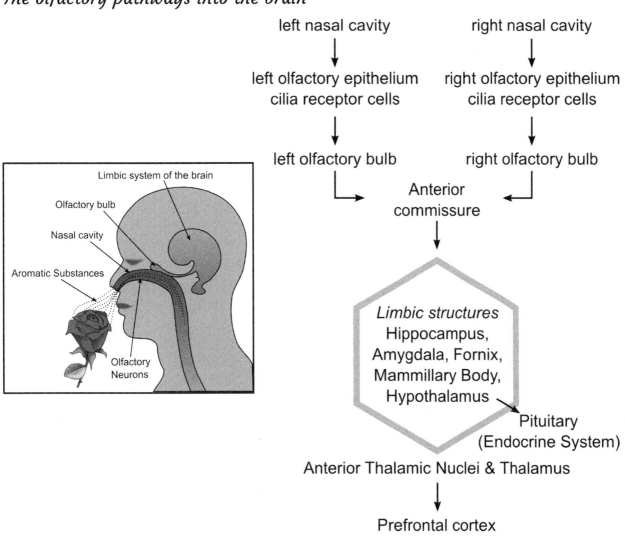

left nasal cavity   right nasal cavity

↓   ↓

left olfactory epithelium   right olfactory epithelium
cilia receptor cells   cilia receptor cells

↓   ↓

left olfactory bulb   right olfactory bulb

→ Anterior commissure ←

↓

Limbic structures
Hippocampus, Amygdala, Fornix, Mammillary Body, Hypothalamus

Pituitary (Endocrine System)

Anterior Thalamic Nuclei & Thalamus

↓

Prefrontal cortex

Labels within figure:
Limbic system of the brain
Olfactory bulb
Nasal cavity
Aromatic Substances
Olfactory Neurons

Chemical molecules exuding from an essential oil, or from essential oils contained within and released from oil glands in flowers and plants, readily combine with oxygen molecules within the surrounding atmosphere as they evaporate. Essential oil molecules are carried within the inflow of air during breathing; oxygen-rich air impregnated with essential oil molecules is drawn up into the nasal cavities, reaching and sweeping across the **olfactory epithelium** situated at the top, or roof, of each cavity, before being redirected down the trachea (windpipe) into the lungs, where the process of gaseous exchange takes place.

Odorant molecules carried within inhaled air are deposited and dissolve in the mucous lining, which acts as a solvent, where they are detected according to their molecular shape by the correspondingly shaped cilia receptor cells (something like a key and lock). Cilia receptor cells have the capacity to provide a matrix of complex combinations (the 'matrix effect') that facilitate increased capacity for detection of multiple odour nuances (something like the way six lottery numbers can be combined in different sequences to form millions of potential numerical combinations). On making contact with odorant molecules, neurons in the cilia convert (transduce) receptor activation into electrical signals, or impulses, that are relayed to and along the olfactory nerve to **mitral cells** in the olfactory bulb. Mitral cells in turn transmute (change) the electrical impulses they receive and relay neural signals from olfactory bulb axons along the olfactory tracts to target receptive areas within the brain that collectively form the **limbic area** or system (sometimes also referred to as the '**emotional brain**') and which includes structures such as the **hypothalamus**, the **amygdala** and the **hippocampus**.

The **pituitary gland** and the hypothalamus are functionally connected to each other through attachment via the pituitary stalk. In spite of this interface, the pituitary gland (the **master endocrine gland**) does not form part of the limbic system. However, when we experience emotions, for example joy or fear, these instigate the hypothalamus to influence the pituitary gland, which then releases hormones that may affect blood pressure or stimulate the heart etc. The pituitary gland is directly involved with metabolic and physiological hormone induced functions and processes, such as growth, regulation of blood pressure, sex organ function, thyroid gland function, water balance via the kidneys, temperature control, pain relief and the metabolic conversion of food into energy.

The olfactory journey within the brain

Electrical signals fired from mitral cells within the olfactory bulbs travel along olfactory tract axons until these converge at the **anterior commissure**. This is situated centrally beneath the frontal cortex in front of the columns of the fornix at the front edge of the 'Limbic area', central to and connecting the left and right hemispheres of the brain. The left and right nasal cavities and olfactory tracts are completely separate until reaching this point. The limbic system comprises four major components, which form two C-shaped structures - one made up of the **hippocampus** and the **fornix**, the other made up of the **cingulate nucleus** and **parahippocampal gyri**. It operates by influencing and stimulating the endocrine system and autonomic nervous system.

Limbic structures associated with identifying odour, such as the amygdala and hippocampus, developed in primitive vertebrates to provide sensory signals to assist their survival (identifying food, mates, predators, dangerous chemicals exuding from rotting or noxious substances etc.); the term '**old brain**' is often ascribed to areas closest to the brain stem and mid brain where these structures are situated. Reaching from structures contained within the primitive sections of the brain to the forebrain cortex (which forms part of 'new mammalian' brain regions), the limbic system is directly connected to the **prefrontal cortex** (situated in the frontal lobe) via signals relayed by dopaminergic neurotransmitters from the **thalamus**. Dopamine is a chemical released by nerve cells to send signals to other nerve cells which are found in the brain and other parts of the body. The prefrontal cortex is where the brain 'makes sense of', identifies, rationalizes, reasons, categorises, decides, in relation to emotional and instinctual messages received from the limbic system (and other sensory systems such as sight, hearing and touch). It is where long term memories are formed.

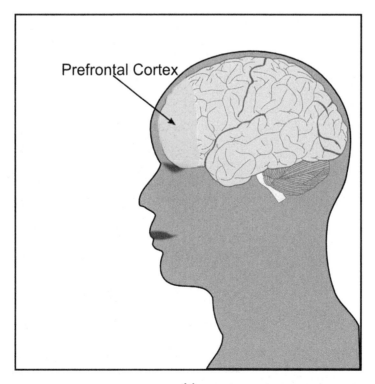

Structures within the limbic system engage multilaterally, instantly generating a complex cluster of interactive psycho-emotional, physiological and behavioural responses. Thus, it is very difficult to absolutely attribute, beyond general indication, specific psycho-emotional actions or to solely attribute these actions to one specific brain region, hormone or function; there are so many variables at play, which are virtually impossible to disentangle from each other. Essential oils are, consequently, generally therapeutically classified under umbrella-terms such as 'stimulating', 'sedating', 'relaxant' etc. However, many essential oils actually possess both stimulating and sedating properties (for example, bergamot, chamomile, clary sage, geranium, lavender, marjoram, patchouli, ylang ylang), while others are 'more sedating'/'less stimulating', 'more stimulating'/'less sedating', rather than being purely one or the other.

Once absorbed into the body's system, essential oils appear to selectively target their action(s) to support or restore physical and psycho-emotional balance, stimulate the immune system and act against pathogens. According to Damian & Damian (1995 p 149) "essential oils… act to heterolaterally harmonize the brain hemispheres" and are psycho-actively more quickly effective, even in small doses, when absorbed via inhalation. Indeed, there are numerous studies (mainly conducted by or on behalf of the food and manufacturing, cosmetic and pharmaceutical industries) exploring the psychotherapeutic effects of essential oils on attention, concentration, productivity, mental-emotional stimulation and sedation, mood states (anxiety, depression, agitation, restlessness), memory and insomnia.

Studies using animals, such as mice, although ethically controversial, eliminate many potentially influential subjective psycho-emotional variables when exploring the basic physiological and behavioural effects of essential oils, and provide very useful indications. However, these studies do not completely reflect the real complexities of true 'life' scenarios when applied to humans, where the idiosyncratic psycho-emotional and hedonistic responses to essential oils contribute to the outcome of their actions; and/or, for that matter, conversely, the complex influence essential oils actually have on the individual's psyche, cognition and physiological function (the inside-out, outside-in response).

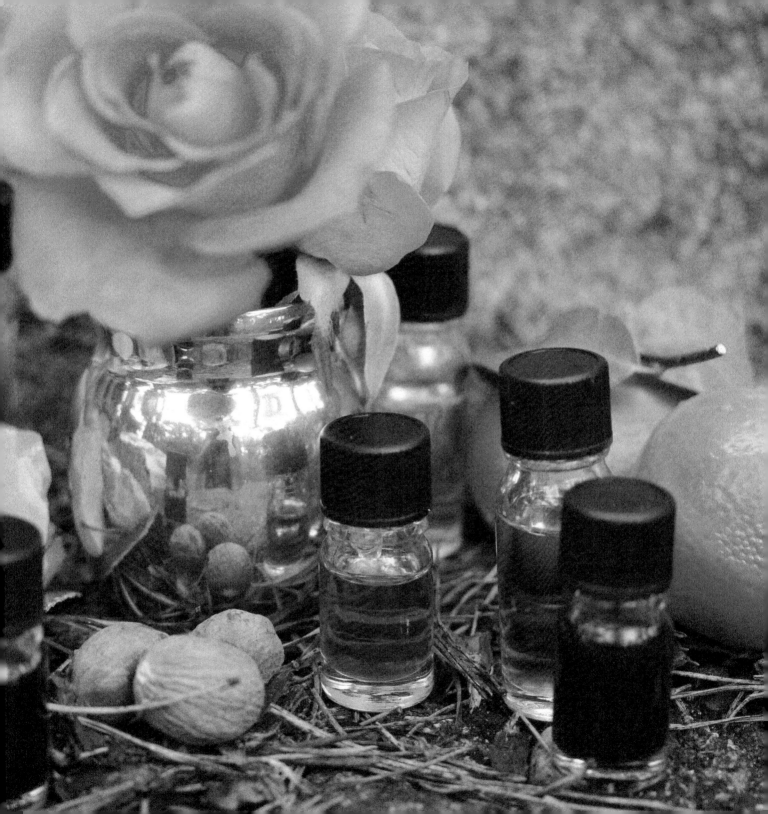

Exploring the psycho-emotional and physiological effects of essential oils

In a study testing the ability of essential oils to calm motility (spontaneous movement) in mice, Buchbauer et al (1993) confirmed the sedative effects of lavender, neroli (orange blossom), linalool, linalyl acetate (isolated chemical components) and citronella when inhaled at low concentration (blood samples revealed the absorption of fragrance compounds), and concluded that "the results contribute to the correct interpretation of the term 'aromatherapy' (i.e. a stimulating or sedative effect on the behavior of individuals upon inhalation of fragrance compounds)". Kovar et al (1987) demonstrated the sedative effect of rosemary essential oil when testing the locomotor activity of mice after inhalation of rosemary, which they attributed in particular to 1,8-cineole, a component of rosemary detected in blood samples post exposure.

In another study involving 144 human subjects, Moss et al (2003) compared the effects of essential oils of rosemary and lavender in one subject group and no essential oil in the control group, to test memory and mental alertness. The participants were aware of the task they were performing, but were not aware that essential oils formed part of the study. The essential oils were diffused into the environment while recipients were engaged in various cognitive tasks. They found that essential oils of lavender (Lavandula angustifolia) and rosemary (Rosmarlnus officinalis) significantly affected aspects of cognition performance.

Lavender decreased the performance of working memory, impairing alertness and retention time for both memory and attention based tasks, while rosemary improved the quality and speed of working memory and secondary memory, and increased alertness; both lavender and rosemary reportedly also produced feelings of contentment during tasks. In a subsequent smaller study, Moss and Oliver (2012) reiterated this finding when testing for speed, accuracy and evaluation of mood during mathematical tasks where 22 subjects were exposed to rosemary essential oil, observing correlation between the higher levels of 1,8-cineole (a chemical component of rosemary found in blood samples post test) and improved performance.

Ilmberger et al (2001), however, found no significant difference in terms of core attentional function in the presence of essential oils, but did observe complex correlation between subjective evaluation of substances and objective task performance. This consequently led to their suggestion that the effects of essential oils (in this case, peppermint, jasmine and ylang ylang) or their components (1,8-cineole, menthol) on basic forms of attentional behavior are actually mainly psychological, and that a subject's expectation of an odour may affect motivation and subsequent behavior, even when merely suggestive.

Friedman (2001), however, examined the effectiveness of essential oils of lavender

(Lavandula angustifolia), cedarwood (Cedrus atlantica) and vetivert (Vetiveria zizanioides,), which were applied to improve the focus and attention of children aged between six and fourteen years diagnosed as presenting with ADHD (Attention Deficit Hyperactive Disorder). EEG (electro-encephalograph) equipment was used to measure beta and theta brain wave activity in areas of the brain before and after a thirty day period of exposure to one of the three essential oils - subjects were asked to inhale, holding the open bottle next to the nostrils and taking three deep breaths, three times per day. The results demonstrated significant improvement in brain activity and reduction of symptoms of ADHD for vetivert (100%), slightly less for cedarwood (83%) and no apparent improvement for lavender (53%), supporting Moss et al's 2003 experimental finding.

Ballard et al (2002) found that melissa (lemon balm) essential oil, when added to a base lotion and applied twice a day to the arms and faces of 72 elderly subjects with severe dementia, significantly improved their agitation - the placebo group received the same treatment, using sunflower oil in place of the melissa (lemon balm) in the lotion. Although this treatment was applied in a topical lotion to the skin, subjects were also exposed to inhalation of the melissa because the lotion was applied to the face, therefore, 'under their noses'.

Burns and Perry (2009) conducted a randomized clinical trial comparing melissa (lemon balm) essential oil, an inactive essential oil (not specified) and the commonly used anti-dementia drug Aricept, and found that melissa significantly decreased agitation in dementia patients. They subsequently undertook further research identifying and confirming that melissa "acts on the brain in two ways, to calm excitatory (serotonin) pathways and stimulate other calming (GABA) pathways" (alzheimers.org.uk/2014). Perry (2014), in a review examining the effectiveness of aromatherapy for the treatment of dementia, reported that lavender, geranium and mandarin blended in sweet almond oil and applied to the skin of elderly patients (again, considering the effects of inhalation) increased their alertness, contentment and ability to sleep at night, and reduced levels of agitation, withdrawal and wandering.

Perry also reported that ylang ylang, patchouli, rosemary and peppermint essential oils significantly decreased disturbed behavior in the majority of the participating dementia patients, which enabled reduction of prescribed medication. In another study, Pengelly et al (2012) found that rosemary (in dried, powdered, herbal form) when consumed orally in low dose (750 mg) similar to its usual culinary consumption, improved the speed of memory in 28 elderly subjects (average age 75 years), but that at high dose (6,000 mg) it significantly impaired memory function (thus highlighting also that the dose, or quantity, is significant for the whole herb and essential oil extracted from the herb). Speed of memory is used as an indicator of impaired cognitive function in the elderly when testing for

Alzheimer's disease or dementia.

Haze et al (2002) investigated the effects of inhalation on sympathetic nervous system activity in normal adult subjects, measuring blood pressure and plasma catecholamine levels from blood samples. Results showed that "inhalation of essential oils, such as black pepper oil, estragon oil, fennel oil or grapefruit oil, resulted in a 1.5 to 2.5-fold increase in relative sympathetic activity, compared with inhalation of an odorless solvent (triethyl citrate)" and, "in contrast, fragrant inhalation of rose oil or patchouli oil caused a 40% decrease in relative sympathetic activity", concluding that "fragrance inhalation of essential oils may modulate sympathetic activity in normal adults."

In a more recent double-blind, placebo controlled clinical study which evaluated the perception of post surgery pain in children aged 3 to 6 years old, Marofi et al (2013) observed significant reduction in pain after diffusion of rose (Rosa damascena Mill.). 64 children (with the consent of their parent or guardian, and ethical clearance from the hospital's clinical research department) were randomly divided into two groups ('A' and 'B'). The children in group 'A' were given the essential oil (rose) and the children in group 'B' sweet almond. Both groups otherwise received exactly the same prescribed post-surgical care.

A post-operative pain assessment (TPPPS –Toddler Preschooler Postoperative Pain Scale) was carried out immediately the children were submitted to their ward. Then an eye pad infused with one or two drops of either rose essential oils or sweet almond oil was placed 30 cm from the child's head. The pain assessment was repeated at 3, 6, 9 and 12 hours after surgery. Although there was initially little difference between both groups after the first assessment, and although there was some reduction of post-operative pain in both groups over the test period, the subsequent assessments did reveal significant decrease in the average score of pain intensity for the essential oil group.

Jellinek (1999, 1997) suggests that "the pharmacological mechanism is far less dominant when it comes to affecting psychological states" and that psychodynamic odour effects, although difficult to prove conclusively, may be based on:

- A quasi-pharmacological mechanism influencing the central nervous system or hormonal systems.
- A semantic mechanism accounting for the influence of personal experiences with certain odours.
- A hedonic valence mechanism providing the dimension for pleasantness for emotional states.
- A placebo mechanism which is based on subjective expectation.

Influencing factor	Pharmacological	Semantic	Hedonistic	Placebo
Biological	●		●	
Personal Experience		●	●	●
Cultural Experience		●	●	●
Personality				●
Olfactory acuity		●		
Stimulus characteristic	chemical	odour	odour	reputation

Jellinek (1999 p 118)

The brain is responsive to external sensory input and neurological stimulation, and facilitates internal homeostasis, environmental awareness, consciousness of a deeper 'sense' of 'being' and relationships with other people and the external 'world'. Fragrance detection triggers numerous neurological, physiological, emotional and hedonistic responses at the same time, which are difficult to disentangle. While it may be very difficult to prove or explain specifically how essential oils affect the brain, as the above studies demonstrate, their vapourising odorous molecules do instigate (to varying degrees) neurological responses that appear to affect mood, emotion, memory, concentration and cognition (either via inhalation or circulatory absorption), even if this influence is only temporary. Meanwhile, research and deliberation continues in a quest for better understanding.

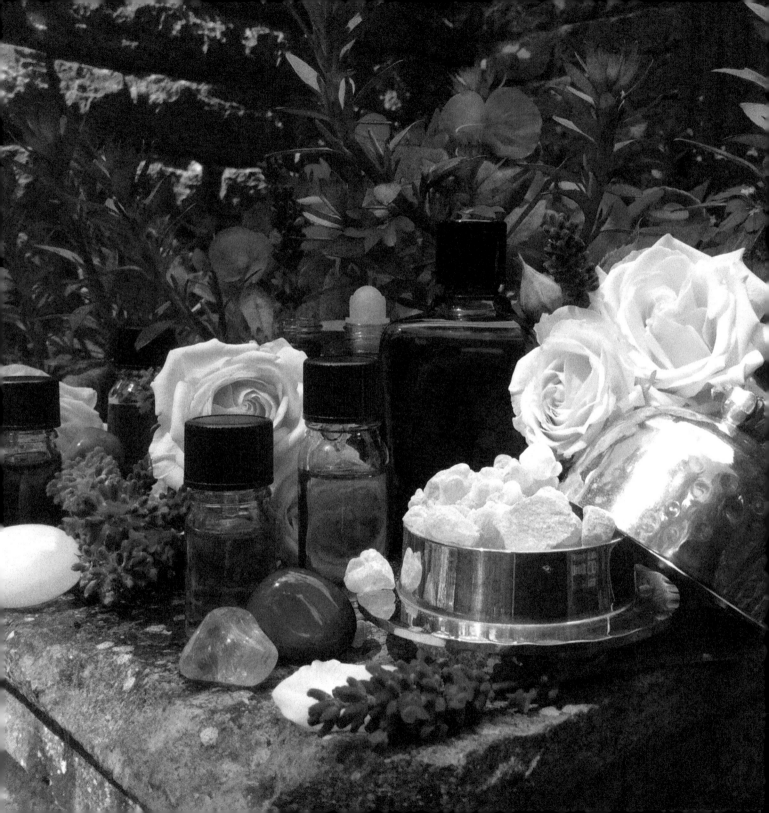

Memory

Odour memory is more tenacious compared with other senses (sight, sound, touch, hearing). Memory is reinforced, enhanced and may last or linger longer where multiple sensory stimulation occurs at the same time, especially when less consciously controlled cognitive processes, which do not involve judgment, deliberation, reasoning or rational evaluation, are being performed; for example, creative tasks, learning and/or performing by rote, etc. (this works the same for negative and positive experiences). Thus, activities such as massage, meditation, visualization or relaxation techniques may be positively enhanced and experientially memorably reinforced when complementary essential oils are vapourised at the same time (and vice versa).

Herz et al (2000) applied odour in connection with pleasant and unpleasant circumstances to examine the effect of odour on memory, finding that "memories elicited by odours are more emotionally potent than memories evoked by other sensory stimuli, and when salient emotion is experienced during odour exposure, the effectiveness of an odour memory cue is enhanced". Pitman (2000) exploited this salient connection between odour and memory to help hyperactive children manage their restlessness, using visualization and self massage during exposure to selected essential oils to instill a sense of calmness and peace that could be recalled and experienced later when deliberately inhaling the odour of the same essential oil(s) as a memory cue, applied and used to calm their behavior and assist their focus on tasks. Pitman observed that, "it was very noticeable that both the oils and the relaxation improved concentration. Students definitely stayed calmer longer and recovered quickly from upsets. There were fewer disruptions to lessons."

Functions of the right and left brain hemispheres

The human brain is separated into two hemispheres, the left and right, which are connected by the corpus callosum which facilitates inter-hemispheric communication. Apparently the left hemisphere of the brain pertains to more logical thought processes and brain activity, and the right hemisphere to more creative. Physiologically, the left hemisphere controls neurological activity to the right side of the body, and the right hemisphere controls neurological activity to the left side of the body. This includes muscle control. Evidence indicates that the left hemisphere is more involved when routine or well rehearsed processing is required and the right hemisphere is more involved in processing new situations. However, brain injury studies demonstrate that both hemispheres have equal capacity to facilitate most processes when neural pathways are redirected to undamaged parts of the brain, although there are exceptions depending on the nature and location of the damage (damage to the hippocampus, for example, can lead to irreversible long-term inability to create new memories).

Left brain processing	Right brain processing
Analytical thought	3-D images
Components	Abstract meaning
Detail	Art awareness
Grammar	Creativity
Language	Expressiveness
Literal meaning	Face recognition
Logic	Hedonistic
Math/number skills	Holistic thought
Name recall	Imagination
Patterns	Insight
Present & past	Intuition
Rational	Music awareness
Reasoning	Philosophy and religion
Safe	Pictures
Science	Practical
Sequential control	Present and future
Theory	Risk taking
Time awareness	Spatial awareness
Words	Spontaneous
Written	Visual imagery
Masculine	Feminine
Yang	Yin

'Gem' Essential oils that potentially have a pronounced influence on certain limbic system structures

Structure	Latin name	Common name
Pituitary	*Pogostemon cablin*	Patchouli
	Rosa damascena / centifolia	Rose
Hypothalamus	*Boswellia carterii*	Frankincense
	Pelargonium asperum / graveolens	Geranium
Anterior Thalamus	*Rosa damascena / centifolia*	Rose
Amygdala & Hippocampus	*Pelargonium asperum / graveolens*	Geranium

Essential Oil	Potential Characteristic Psycho-emotional Action and Support	Potential Associated Limbic Structure
Cajeput *(Melaleuca cajeputii)*	Aids concentration, clears and stimulates the mind, clears thoughts, helps find courage in finding new pathways and managing change, strengthens resolve and 'spirit'	Anterior Thalamus
Galbanum *(Ferula galbaniflua)*	Balancing, both sedative and stimulant, calms erratic moods, nervous tension, menopausal symptoms, pre-menstrual tension (PMT), stress and stress related conditions, tonic, lifts mood and is restorative (nerves)	Hypothalamus
Mandarin *(Citrus reticulata)*	'Awakens', 'brings out' the inner child; good for quelling anxiety, depression and low mood, hyperactivity (although orange can encourage hyperactivity, mandarin is calming), insomnia, nervous tension, panic attacks, pre-menstrual tension (PMT), restlessness, stress and stress related conditions, has a sedative quality	Hypothalamus Amygdala
Petitgrain *(Citrus aurantium var amara)*	Eases anger, anxiety, depression, hyperactivity, insomnia, mental clarity, nervous exhaustion, nervous system sedative, nervous tension, pre-menstrual tension (PMT), sense of hopelessness,	Anterior Thalamus Hypothalamus

	stress and stress related conditions	
Tea tree *(Melaleuca alternifolia)*	Revitalising and stimulating, helpful for apathy, 'cleansing', nervous exhaustion and shock	Anterior Thalamus Hypothalamus
Carrot seed *(Daucus carota)*	Eases anxiety, apathy, calms experience of stress, confusion, inability to 'move on', indecision, mental clarity, mental and emotional exhaustion, nervous system sedative, revitalizing	Anterior Thalamus Hypothalamus
Chamomile German *(Matricaria recutita)*	Eases anxiety, calms experience of stress, headaches, insomnia, migraine, mood swings, nervous tension, pre-menstrual tension (PMT), mental (calms an active mind) and nervous system sedative	Anterior Thalamus Hypothalamus
Chamomile Roman *(Chamaemelum nobilis, Anthemis nobilis)*	Eases anger, anxiety, calms experience of stress, fear, hyperactivity, impatience, insomnia, irritability, pre-menstrual tension (PMT), restlessness, solar plexus tension, mental, emotional and nervous system sedative	Anterior Thalamus Hypothalamus Amygdala
Cypress *(Cupressus sempervirens)*	Eases anger, anxiety, confusion and indecision, dwelling on unpleasant events, grief and bereavement, impatience, inability to 'move on', irritability and intolerance, lack of concentration, nervous tension, pre-menstrual tension (PMT),	Anterior Thalamus Hypothalamus Amygdala / Hippocampus

	regulates autonomic nervous system, stress and stress related conditions, uncontrolled crying, sedative	
Geranium Rose *(Pelargonium graveolens roseum)*	Both sedative and stimulant. Eases anxiety, depression and low mood, headaches, jealousy, nervous tension, menopausal problems, mood swings, neuro-balancing, pre-menstrual tension (PMT), solar plexus balance, stress and stress related conditions, uplifting, endocrine stimulant (hormone-like)	Anterior Thalamus Hypothalamus
Lavender *(Lavandula angustifolia Mill)* *Lavandula vera D.C. ssp.)* **Lavender Spike** *(Lavandula latifolia)*	Sedative at low dose stimulant at high, eases agitation, anger, anxiety, depression, grief and bereavement, headaches, insomnia, irritability and intolerance, manic depression (professional support required), mood swings, nervous tension, panic, pre-menstrual tension (PMT), sense of hopelessness, shock, solar plexus tension, stress and stress related conditions, suspicion	Anterior Thalamus Hypothalamus Amygdala
Frankincense *(Boswellia carterii)*	Eases anger, anxiety, confusion and indecision, depression and low mood, dwelling on unpleasant events, fear and paranoia, grief and bereavement, helps let go of unwanted thoughts and memories, hyperactivity, impatience, inability to 'move on', irritability and intolerance, mood swings, nervous	Anterior Thalamus Hypothalamus Amygdala / Hippocampus

	tension, panic attacks (calms and relaxes breathing), pre-menstrual tension (PMT), resentment and disappointment, sadness and despair, sedative, supports meditation and finding inner tranquility	
Patchouli *(Pogostemon cablin Benth.)*	Sedative at low dose stimulant at high, eases apathy, confusion and indecision, depression and low mood, nervous exhaustion, nervous tension, panic attacks, pre-menstrual tension (PMT), stress and stress related conditions, endocrine stimulant, supports meditation and a sense of 'spirituality'	Anterior Thalamus Hypothalamus
Rose Otto *(Rosa damascena, Rosa centifolia)*	Sedative at low dose stimulant at high, eases agitation, anger, anxiety, depression (especially postnatal) and low mood, fear and paranoia, grief and bereavement (and sense of loss), hatred, headaches (tension and hormonal), hypersensitivity, insomnia, jealousy, migraine, nervous tension, panic attacks, pre-menstrual tension (PMT), resentment and disappointment, sadness and despair, stress and stress related conditions, endocrine stimulant (hormone-like), aphrodisiac	Anterior Thalamus Hypothalamus Amygdala
Spikenard *(Nardostachys jatamansi*	Balances sympathetic nervous system with parasympathetic nervous system (tonic to the	Anterior Thalamus Hypothalamus

D.C. **_Nardostachys grandiflora_** **D.C._)_**	sympathetic nervous system, regulates the parasympathetic nervous system). 'Grounding', eases anxiety, calms restlessness, grief and bereavement, hatred, headaches and migraine, hyperactivity, hysteria, impatience, insomnia, intolerance, irritability, nervous indigestion, nervous tension, panic attacks, PMS, menopausal symptoms, stress and stress related conditions, sedative	
Vetivert **(Vetiveria zizanoides L.** **Stapf.)**	Reduces symptoms of withdrawal when coming off medication (especially tranquillisers), balances the central nervous system, eases anxiety, confusion and indecision, debility, depression, hyperactivity, hypersensitivity, impatience, insomnia, mental exhaustion, nervous system sedative, nervous tension, panic attacks, pre-menstrual tension and menopausal symptoms, stress and stress related conditions, sedative, 'earthing' and 'grounding'	Anterior Thalamus Hypothalamus Amygdala

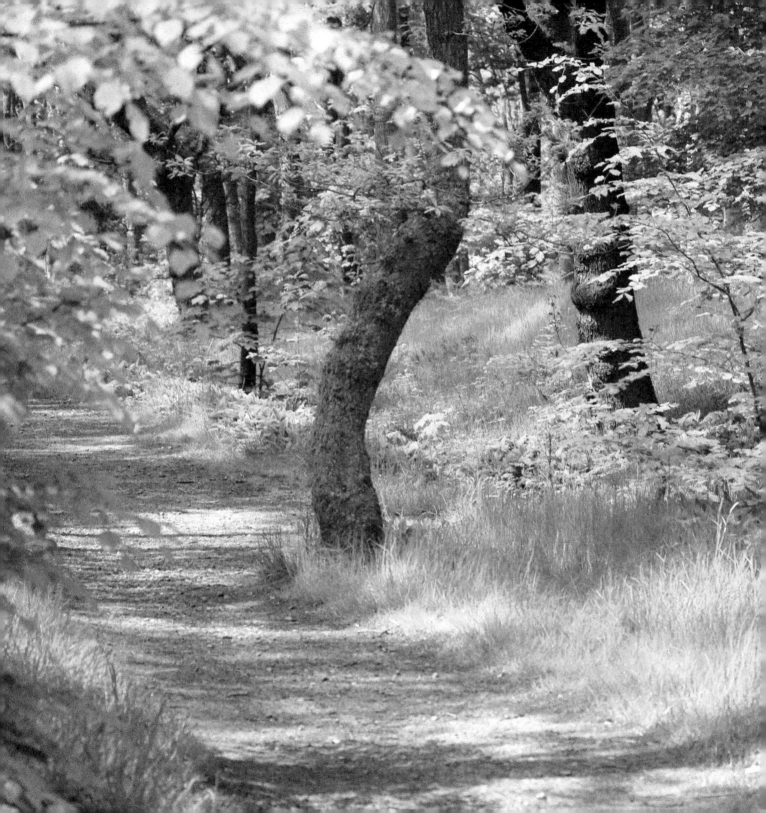

Subjective terms used to describe psycho-emotional effects of essential oils

- Calming
- Bracing
- Grounding
- Warming
- Balancing
- Restorative
- Invigorating
- Refreshing
- Strengthening
- Uplifting

The primary cephalic actions most commonly cited as being supported by essential oils:

- Sedative / Calming
- Stimulant / Uplifting
- Balance of the central nervous system

Psycho-emotional conditions that essential oils may ease:

- Anger
- Anxiety
- Depression
- Fear
- Grief
- Headaches
- Insomnia
- Mental clarity
- Mental exhaustion
- Mood swings
- Nervous tension
- Nervous exhaustion
- Restlessness
- Shock

Odour receptors are expressed in many tissues, not just the olfactory epithelium. They exist throughout the body in organ (for example, liver, heart, kidneys, spleen, colon, lungs, brain and testes) and epidermal tissue, and are able to detect a multitude of compounds. Just as in olfactory detection, odour receptors detect molecules (lock-key) and in turn trigger and relay neural signals, which activate a cellular response. For example, odour receptors in the kidneys help control metabolic function and regulate blood pressure. Odour cells within the testes aid fertilization through attraction, guiding the sperm cell to the ovulated egg. Keratinocytes, the major cells of the epidermis, contain olfactory receptors; odour molecules stimulate these cells, affecting cell proliferation and migration, and regeneration and rejuvenation – a significant process in wound healing. Discovery of the existence of odour cells beyond the olfactory epithelium, however, is relatively recent and further research is required to identify the extent of the function of these cells. This discovery is, none-the-less, very significant in terms of the application of essential oils and helps to explain the healing, regenerating and rejuvenating properties, among others, of essential oils. (Busse et al 2014; Stone 2014; Griffin 2009; Pluznick 2008; Spehr 2003)

The Lungs

Passing through the nose, across the olfactory epithelium, oxygen rich air containing essential oil molecules continues its journey down the trachea (wind pipe), into the bronchi (tubes entering the lungs), then into the lung cavity, where gaseous exchange takes place, facilitated by the alveoli (tiny specialized hollow air sacs found at the end of alveolar ducts and atria). The thin porous membrane surrounding each alveolus contains a matrix, or network, of pulmonary arterial and venal capillaries, which facilitate the movement of oxygen and carbon dioxide between air and blood. Oxygen, along with other air-borne molecules, such as those from essential oils, diffuses from the inhaled air momentarily contained within the lungs into the arterial capillaries, from where the oxygen infused blood travels away from the lungs (through arterioles and arteries) via the circulatory system to cells throughout the body; thus essential oil molecules are carried via the blood into the internal organs and cells. The cells in exchange release carbon dioxide (CO_2) into the blood which is carried from organs and other tissues via veins then ultimately into venal alveolar capillaries where, along with other blood-borne volatile compounds, CO_2 diffuses out through the thin porous membrane surface into the air still held momentarily within the lungs, before being excreted from the body via exhalation of the breath. Each lung contains around 350 million alveoli, which collectively provide approximately 70 to 100 square meters of surface area! A certain amount of gaseous diffusion also takes place within the capillary lined nasal cavity, pharynx and mucous membrane en route to the lungs.

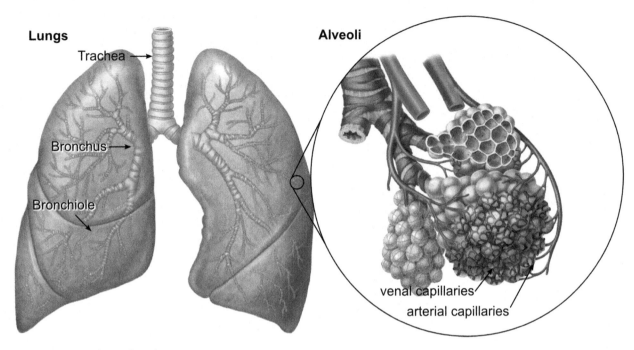

Lungs
Trachea
Bronchus
Bronchiole

Alveoli
venal capillaries
arterial capillaries

Essential oil characteristics

Description	Top Note	Middle Note	Base Note
Type of oils	Lemon and other citrus fruits; leaves	Herbs; flowering tops	Resins, woods, roots, blossoms
Therapeutic Effects	Uplifting, stimulating, cephalic, revitalising	'Balancing', harmonizing, rejuvenating	Relaxing, 'earthing', sedating, calming
May support / ease (general indications)	Extreme lethargy, melancholy, lack of interest, apathy, depression, acute	Bodily functions, metabolism, digestion, menstruation, circulation (blood pressure)	Nervous, erratic or flighty, hyperactive. Chronic and/or long standing conditions, the elderly, anxiety
Action	Fast	Moderate	Slow
Skin penetration	½ hour to 1 hour	2 hours to 3 hours	4 hours to 6 hours or more

Evaporation rate	0 to 30 minutes	Up to 8 hours	Up to 12 to 24 hours, a week, sometimes longer
Volatility rate Scale 1 to 100	*Most volatile* 1 to 14	15 to 60	*Least volatile* 61 to 100
General odour Characteristic	Sharpish	'Round', 'soft edges'	Heavy, rich, intense
Evaporation and 'dry out' odour behaviour and characteristics	Fresh, distinctive, cluster of odours, obvious, light, potentially intense due to rapid evaporation.	Lingering traces of top notes; heart of the bouquet, the character; 'softer' edges (not 'sharp')	Lingering traces of middle notes, faint, faded, subtle, non-descript; or, heavy, tenacious residue
Essential oils	Cajeput Galbanum Mandarin Petitgrain * Tea tree	Carrot seed Chamomile(s) Cypress * Frankincense* Geranium Lavender Petitgrain* Rose * Spikenard *	Cypress * Frankincense * Patchouli Rose * Spikenard * Vetivert

* top to middle, middle to top – middle to base, base to middle

The odour and therapeutic characteristics and behaviours of some essential oils overlap into adjacent 'notes' (these oils are identified with *) depending on their source (part or type of plant etc), chemical constituents and volatility rate (general categorisation sometimes differs between authors). To maintain a link between the fast and slow elements (top and base), and to reduce rapid evaporation of more volatile components, include at least one middle note in all blends.

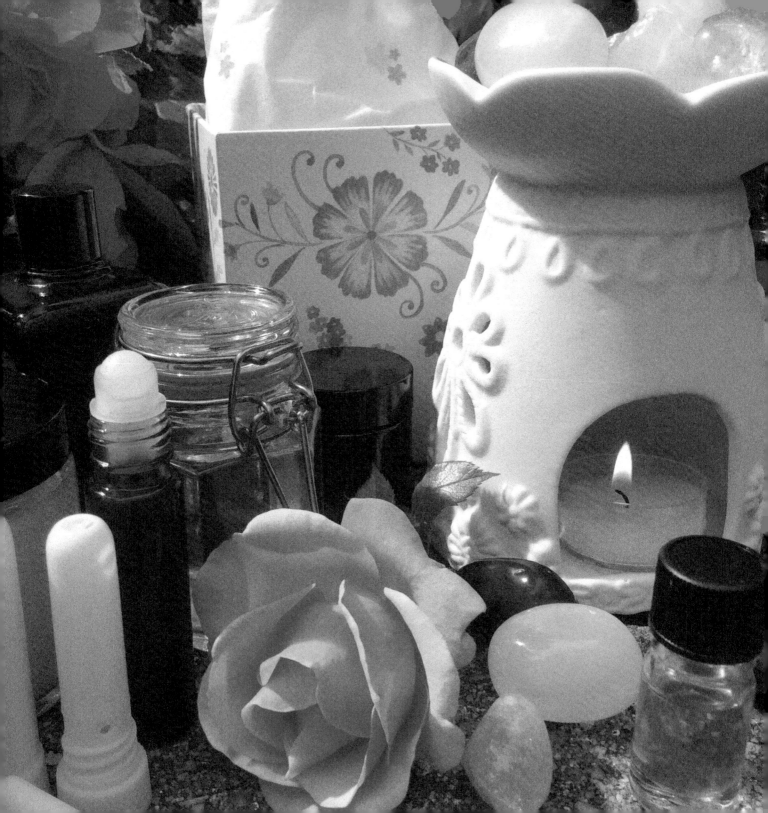

Methods of Use and Application

Safe Application

I do not advocate the internal use of essential oils here, or in any of the books in the Aromantique compilation, unless prescribed by a professional practitioner with biomedical, pharmaceutical or herbalist training; awareness of the chemical interaction and physiological effects of essential oils is imperative. Essential oils are highly concentrated, volatile, odiferous chemicals, with propensity to cause irritation and sensitization and for some people, although relatively rare, allergic reaction, if not applied appropriately. Aromantique's Essential Oil Gems: Absorption, Characteristics and Application, provides a sound background understanding of the nature and safe use of essential oils.

Purchasing Essential Oils

Firstly, ensure that you purchase essential oils from a reputable supplier whose oils are fresh, correctly packaged and appropriately labelled, and who can vouch for the integrity of the oils they supply (details of the source, location of growth, botanical family, Latin name, batch number, safety data information and so on). Oils that are much cheaper than average are potentially not genuine and are often adulterated or bulked out with inferior, less expensive chemicals (equally, very expensive essential oils are often adulterated with cheaper substitute chemicals or essential oils to increase profit margins). Read the labels carefully to ensure that bottles or products contain 100% pure essential oils. Also, only purchase essential oils stored in amber or blue glass bottles (to protect against UV light damage) with a dropper cap (this ensures careful measurement, inhibits rapid oxidization, prevents spillage and limits accidental ingestion by children - ask for child proof lids if necessary). Never purchase or use essential oils that have been stored in plastic bottles and do not purchase essential oils that have been stored on brightly lit, warm shelves. Essential oils are highly flammable so should be kept away from fire (candles etc.) and sources of intense heat.

Secondly, ensure that you know about the chemical and therapeutic properties of and applicable contra-indications and cautions in relation to the essential oil(s) you intend to apply before use.

Methods of Use

There are various methods of applying essential oils. When applied appropriately, essential oils pose little risk; however, while their therapeutic qualities are undoubtedly highly beneficial, they are best used in limited, controlled amounts, especially when applying them on a frequent or daily basis. As a general rule, 6 drops of essential oil per day is the appropriate, safe limit applied for epidermal (perfume, massage, cream, lotion, ointment) or direct olfactory absorption (steam inhalation or smelling strip). I have observed through my therapeutic practice that, even when applied in very small amounts, essential oils can procure a very effective response. **It is very important to measure essential oils carefully, as they are prone to cause skin and mucous membrane irritation and sensitivity if over used or inappropriately applied**.

The following information applies to the use of essential oils as companions for mindfulness. For further information about methods of applying essential oils, please refer to **Aromantique's Essential Oil Gems: Absorption, Characteristics and Application.**

Essential Oils – Cautions to observe

- Do not apply essential oils neat on the skin (always dilute in a vegetable oil, non-perfumed lotion or cream) – undiluted dermal application of essential oils can lead to irritation and sensitisation. Lavender and tea tree essential oils are the exception to this rule (often used as a first aid remedy for insect stings, minor burns or skin abrasions, or mild skin infections), but repeated long term topical application of these oils is not advisable due to the risk of sensitisation.
- Do not swallow or take essential oils internally.
- Keep out of the reach of children (suppliers will provide child proof lids if requested) and away from pets.
- Accidental ingestion: DO NOT INDUCE VOMITING. Drink full fat milk. Seek medical advice immediately. Keep the bottle the essential oil was stored in for identification (label should have Latin name, batch no., sell-by date etc., the bottle will have traces of the oil).
- Eyes: Essential oils can be transferred from fingers to the eyes (always wash your hands after using or handling essential oils). If NEAT essential oil enters your eyes IMMEDIATELY flush with vegetable oil or full fat milk, then rinse thoroughly with clean, warm water. Sometimes diluted essential oils enter the eyes during steam inhalation, bathing or showering, if this happens immediately flush eyes with clean warm water. In either case, seek medical advice IMMEDIATELY if irritation or stinging

persists after flushing the eye(s).

- Skin reaction: Apply vegetable oil to dilute the essential oil on the skin, then thoroughly wash the area with non-perfumed soap (liquid soap if possible) and rinse with warm water to remove any trace of soap and the essential oil. Dry the area thoroughly and apply a non-perfumed base cream (vegetable oil or even butter if nothing else is available) to soothe irritation if appropriate.
- Only purchase from reputable suppliers (who will provide safety data information).
- Only purchase essential oils stored in amber or dark blue glass bottles with 'dropper top' lids (to ensure careful measurement, prevent spillage or accidental ingestion).
- Check the sell-by date before use and make a note of the date of purchase (essential oils oxidise rapidly when exposed to oxygen in the atmosphere, therefore they have a limited shelf life):
    2 years if unopened
    1 year once opened (citrus oils, such as mandarin, 6 months once opened)
- Never 'top-up' a bottle of essential oil with more essential oil once opened for use.
- Discard small amounts of essential oil left in a bottle or container, unless rapidly used up from the moment of first opening the bottle.
- Replace lids immediately after use (to slow down oxidisation).
- Store in a cool dark place, away from sources of heat and direct sunlight (preferably a fridge – some oils, such as rose Otto, however, will solidify when very cold, but will return to a liquid state at room temperature).
- Wipe up spillages immediately (essential oils will dissolve / damage polystyrene, plastic, varnish, paint, polished and laminated surfaces).

Methods of Application

General Guidelines

Decide on your specific purpose or theme to hone your essential oil selection, for example, to aid relaxation, to stimulate alertness, to create a particular ambiance, to aid a particular emotion (uplifting, grounding, balancing), to aid meditation and so on.

It's OK to use a single specially selected essential oil – a single well chosen essential oil can be as equally effective as a blend of essential oils.

If you decide to use more than one essential oil in a blend, limit this to three or four essential oils and affirm their compatibility, or harmony, with each other.

When using more than one essential oil aim to include different 'notes' to enhance the balance and tenacity of your blend (remember, base 'note' essential oils linger longest, top 'notes' evaporate very quickly).

Avoid blending stimulating essential oils with relaxing essential oils.

Avoid using the same essential oil or blend of essential oils repeatedly. Change your selection from time to time. If using essential oils regularly for their psycho-emotional qualities, apply reduced amounts - 'less is more' when applying over long periods of time.

Take breaks of abstinence. For example, use your essential oils for three or four weeks than have a week's break. Changing the essential oil and changing the blended combinations you use will aid in avoiding sensitisation to a particular essential oil or chemical component(s) found within oil(s) applied.

Stop using your selected essential oil or essential oil blend immediately if you feel nauseous, develop a headache or skin rash, redness or itchiness (particularly at the point of application).

If vapourising essential oils in a communal or public area ensure those people sharing the area agree / are aware that you are doing so. Do not take for granted that everyone likes the odour of essential oils or those essential oils you like and select.

Measuring Essential Oils

Measurement percentages can seem quite complicated, especially considering that dropper top sizes vary, rendering absolute accuracy impossible. However, in the interest of safety, essential oil quantities do need to be monitored. Therefore, as a 'rule of thumb guide', assume the averages set out in the measurement guide below.

Risk of sensitivity or irritation reactions increases where large amounts of essential oil are applied to very small areas of skin – applying 6 drops of essential oil in a carrier medium to the whole body through massage will have negligible irritant effect, yet the same quantity of essential oil applied to a small area of skin can be irritant, particularly in sensitive areas such as the face, under arms etc.

Use no more than 1 or 2 drops of essential oils in a carrier medium on localized areas of skin. Keep this in mind when making first aid ointments or face creams or lotions. When making face creams etc. for regular use, reduce the amount of essential oils included, change the essential oil selection from time to time, and have 'no essential oil' breaks in between use.

Measurement Guide

5 ml (bottle) = 100 drops of essential oil.

10 ml (bottle) = 200 drops of essential oil

Maximum amount of essential oil per 24 hour period = 6 to 10 drops (healthy adult – see below). Apply for 2 to 3 weeks only, followed by 1 week's abstinence, and change essential oil(s) selection regularly.

Carrier Medium = vegetable oils, creams, lotions, oitments, gels

- 1 drop of essential oil in 5 ml of carrier medium = 1% blend
- 2 ½ drops of essential oil in 5 ml of carrier medium = 2.5% blend
- 5 drops of essential oil in in 5 ml of carrier medium = 5% blend

Appropriate quantities

Reduced amount

For children and babies over 3 months old (for babies between 3 months and 24 months old use the maximum dilution), for those who are frail or very elderly and those with sensitivities, allergies, eczema, asthma. Also for facial blends.

- 1 drop of essential oil in 5 ml of carrier medium = 1% blend
- 2 drops of essential oil in 10 ml of carrier medium = 1% blend

- 1 drop of essential oil in 10 ml of carrier medium = 0.5% blend
- 2 drops of essential oil in 20 ml of carrier medium = 0.5% blend

- 1 drop of essential oil in 20ml of carrier medium = 0.25% blend

Normal amount

For general and adult use

- 2 ½ drops of essential oil in 5 ml of carrier medium = 2.5% blend
- 5 drops of essential oil in 10 ml of carrier medium = 2.5% blend

Acute / exceptional amount

For acute, short-term occasional use. Avoid or reduce the use of known irritant oils and use quenching oils in blend.

- 5 drops of essential oil in 5 ml of carrier medium = 5% blend
- 10 drops of essential oil in 10 ml carrier medium = 5% blend

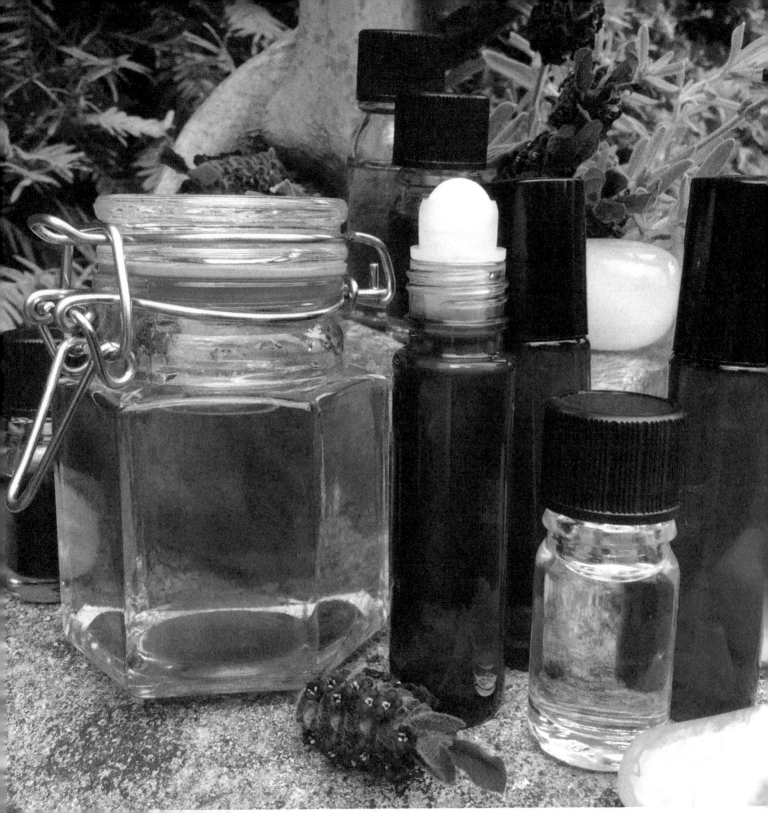

Roller Bottles

Therapeutic and aesthetic perfumes.

Half fill the bottle (usually 10 ml) with a base oil, for example, jojoba oil or other selected vegetable oil(s), for example, borage seed, grapeseed etc. (do not use mineral oil). Add up to 10 drops of your chosen essential oil or blend of essential oils. Top up with base oil to the shoulder of the bottle. Secure roller ball cap and lid. Roll the bottle rapidly between the palms and fingers of your hands to 'shake up' and disperse the essential oils throughout the base oil. Leave in a cool place to stand for 24 hours to allow essential oils to diffuse evenly into the base oil. Remove external cap and roll the perfume oil onto wrists or temples as and when required, replacing the lid immediately after use (use within 6 weeks).

NB: For personal application only. The roller bottle can be re-used (and / or recycled) – wash with warm soapy water, rinse and dry thoroughly before refilling (or recycling).

Use for:

- Aesthetic – attractant; mood; occasion; theme.
- Anxiety and depression.
- Headaches.
- Improve, or reinforce, memory retention.
- Psycho-emotional moods and conditions – for example, for grief, joy, loss, nervousness, pleasure; balance, calm, invigorate, sedate, to 'feel good', uplift.
- Stress, stress related conditions.

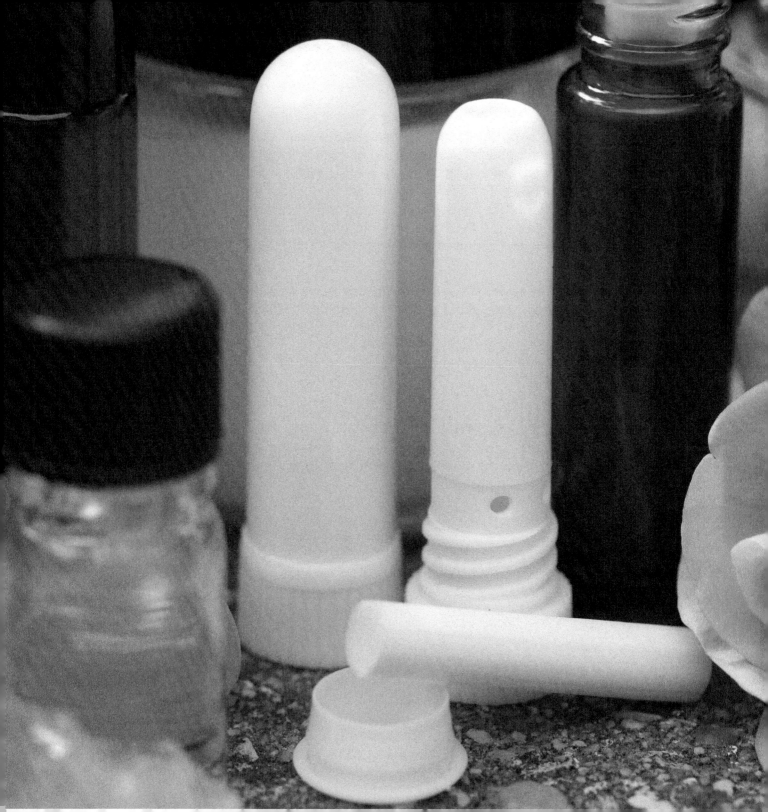

Nasal Inhalers

Therapeutic Inhaler

Dismantle nasal inhaler to remove wadding roll inside the containing tube. Add 2 to 6 drops of your selected essential oil or blend of essential oils to the wadding roll. Replace essential oil infused wadding into the containing tube and secure cover and cap. Remove covering cap and inhale through each nostril as required, replacing cap immediately after use.

NB: for personal application only. The plastic container can be re-used (and / or recycled) – wash with warm soapy water, rinse and dry thoroughly before re-using (or recycling). Replace wadding roll with a roll of cotton wool or tissue.

Use for:

- Anxiety and depression.
- Chest infections.
- Colds and 'flu.
- Headaches.
- Immune support (anti microbial, anti-infectious, anti viral).
- Improve respiration.
- Improve, or reinforce, memory retention.
- Insomnia.
- Mental clarity (to clear head and thoughts).
- Psycho-emotional moods and conditions – for example, for grief, joy, loss, nervousness, pleasure; balance, calm, invigorate, sedate, to 'feel good', uplift.
- Sinus congestion.
- Sore throats.
- Stress, stress related conditions.

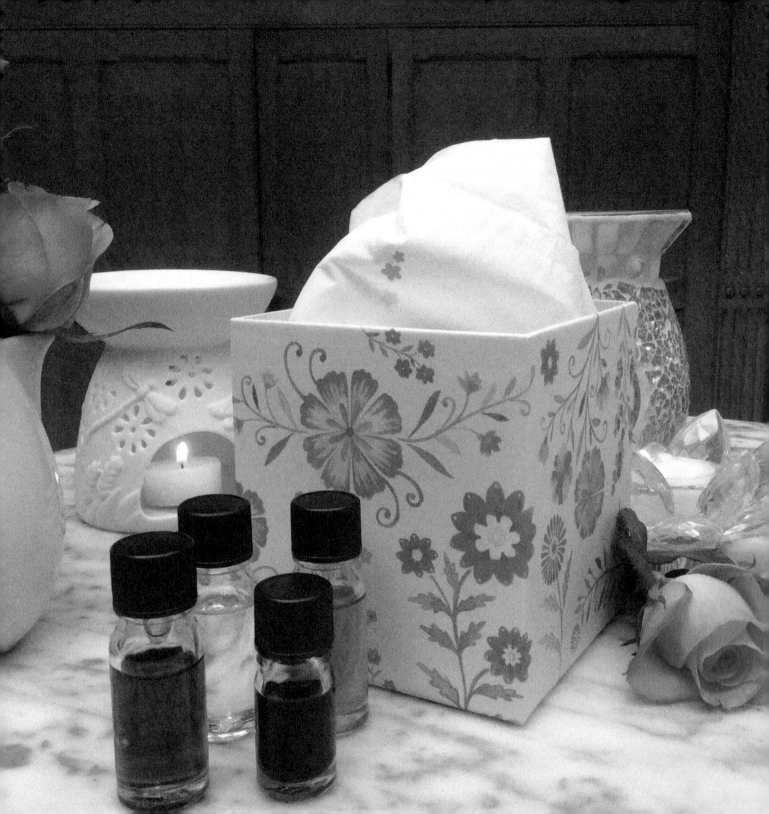

Tissues

Therapeutic inhalation

Add 1 to 3 drops of your selected essential oil or blend of essential oils. Inhale vapours from tissue as required. Do not allow essential oil infused tissue to touch the skin on your face or nose to avoid potential skin irritation.

Useful method for immediate need or for first aid (headaches, shock, upset etc.).

Hold essential oil infused tissue in cupped hands, one hand as base, the other cupped over the palm of this hand forming an enclosed receptacle for the tissue (thus temporarily containing the evaporating vapours), with a small inhaling gap between the thumb and forefinger of the second hand – inhale vapourising odours through the gap created. WASH HANDS WHEN THIS EXERCISE IS FINISHED to remove excess essential oil that may have transferred from the tissue to your hands or fingers.

Use for:
- Anxiety and depression (mild).
- Chest infections.
- Colds and 'flu.
- Headaches.
- Immune support (anti microbial, anti-infectious, anti viral).
- Improve respiration.
- Improve, or reinforce, memory retention.
- Insomnia.
- Mental clarity (to clear head and thoughts).
- Psycho-emotional moods and conditions – for example, for grief, joy, loss, nervousness, pleasure; balance, calm, invigorate, sedate, to 'feel good', uplift.
- Shock and upset.
- Sinus congestion.
- Sore throat.
- Stress, stress related conditions.

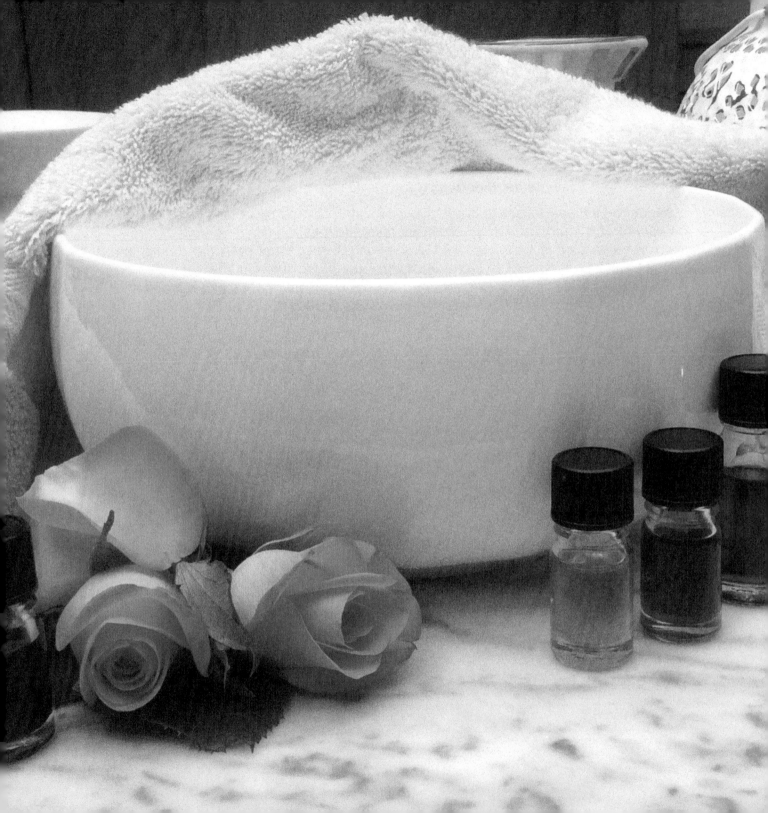

Steam Inhalation

Therapeutic inhalation

You will need: a kettle (or pan), water, bowl, tissues, essential oils and a large towel. Before commencing, ensure that your equipment is placed in a safe position, away from pets and children, and on a stable surface. Heat the water to boiling point. Very carefully pour boiled water from the kettle (or pan) into the bowl (preferably heat proof ceramic, glass or pottery – do not use plastic bowls). Allow the water to cool slightly (essential oils will vapourise too rapidly otherwise). Add 2 to 4 drops of your selected essential oil or blend of essential oils to the water (replace essential oil bottle lids immediately). Cover your head and the bowl with the large towel to contain the rising essential oil infused steam vapours - CLOSE YOUR EYES.

Breath vapours through your nose, exhale through your mouth, for a few minutes. Remove towel ('come up for air'). Replenish water and essential oils if necessary and repeat exercise two or three times. Stop immediately if you experience any irritation or feel dizzy. Essential oils will irritate the mucous membrane to a certain degree; use moderately and do not exceed the above dose. Caution must be applied if the recipient has sensitivities, asthma or epilepsy (half the above dose – 1 to 2 drops of essential oils).

Use for:

- Anxiety and depression (mild).
- Chest or bronchial infections or conditions.
- Headaches, colds and 'flu.
- Immune support (anti microbial, anti-infectious, anti viral).
- Improve respiration.
- Insomnia.
- Loosen and / or encourage expulsion of mucous (expectorant).
- Mental clarity (to clear head and thoughts).
- Psycho-emotional moods and conditions – for example, for grief, joy, loss, nervousness, pleasure; to balance, calm, invigorate, sedate, 'feel good', uplift.
- Sinus congestion.
- Skin care: opening and cleansing pores; acne and oily skin; revitalizing and rejuvenating the facial / neck skin (rinse with cool water and / or witch hazel after steam inhalation procedure to close pores).
- Sore throat.
- Stress, stress related conditions.

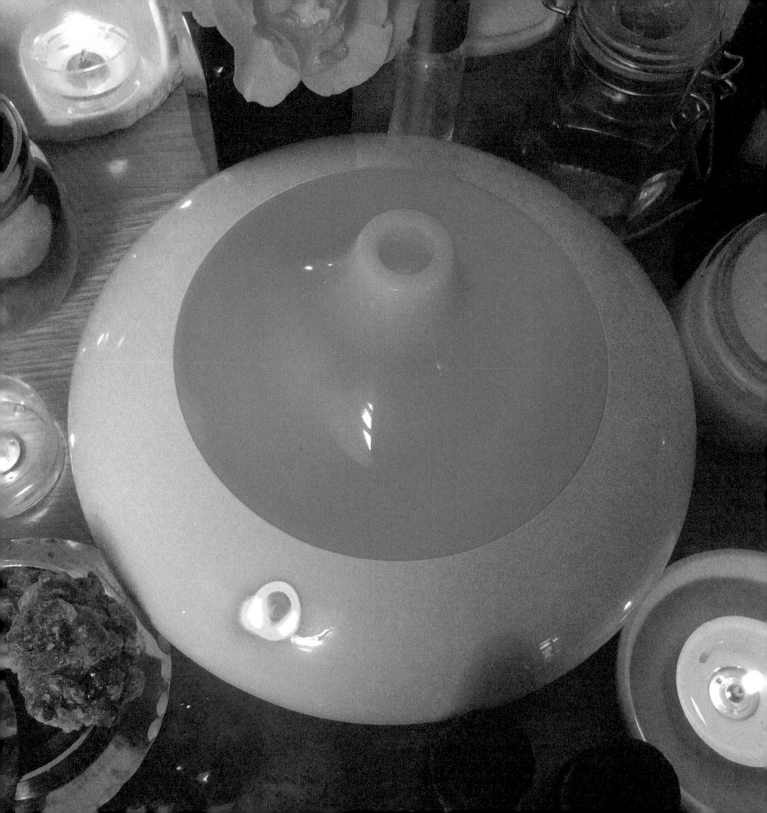

Environmental Room Vapourisers and Diffusers

Candle lit burners are a very popular way of diffusing essential oils and they do create a lovely ambiance. However, care must be taken when using this method; for example, always ensure that the candle is extinguished before leaving the burner unattended, keep out of the reach of children and so on.

Electric steam diffusers have come on in leaps and bounds in terms of their design and are becoming increasingly popular, especially as they are safer to use (although caution must still be applied). These tend to dispense the essential oil infused steam more rapidly and further into the atmosphere of a room and seem to maintain the integrity of the odour better than other methods of diffusion.

Most essential oils can be diffused in either way. However, essential oils extracted from fruits (for example, **mandarin*** and lime), woods (for example, sandalwood, cedarwood, **cypress*** and pine), flowers (for example, ylang ylang, orange blossom and of course **rose***) and resins (such as **frankincense*** and myrrh) to name just a few examples, are especially refreshing, pleasant and tenacious and can be combined to make lovely blends. Rose Otto essential oil is extremely expensive. Rose absolute though, is less so. Either can be purchased in a 5% mix usually blended in jojoba oil. Both the absolute and Otto are intensely perfumed so using a very small amount is still very effective.

Remember, odour preference is very personal and what one person may really like another person may not, so when you diffuse essential oils in a communal area be mindful that the essential oils you choose are agreeable.

The sense of smell soon becomes saturated; the brain stops acknowledging smells after a short period of time, even though they may still be present (leaving and returning to a room, the odour is re-acknowledged; this may be a good indication of whether the essential oils need replenishing).

*'Essential Oil Gems'

Electric fan or steam diffusers

These usually come with instructions regarding appropriate operation and use. Add 6 to 8 drops of an essential oil or essential oil blend. Replenish as necessary. Rather than leaving the diffuser on constantly, use in short 'bursts' at chosen convenient times.

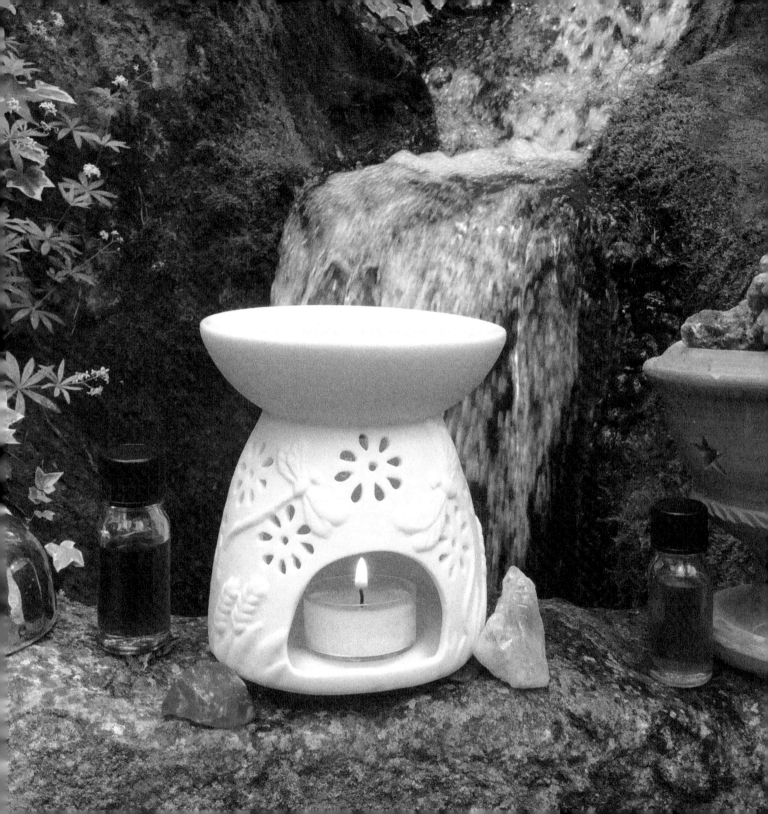

Candle Burners

Add water to the bowl. Add 6 to 8 drops of essential oil or essential oil blend. Light candle. Replenish as necessary. Burners with deep bowls are preferable (to avoid rapid drying out). Do not allow water to dry out (keep a small jug of water at hand to replenish). Do not leave unattended or where they may be knocked over (fire risk); keep out of reach of children and pets.

Uses

- Aesthetic (environmental) perfume.
- Anti-anxiety.
- Anti-depressing.
- Calming.
- Improve and / or support mood and emotion.
- Improve or create a particular ambience or theme.
- Insomnia.
- Mask unpleasant odours.
- Reduce or combat airborne microbes.
- Reduce restlessness and agitation (calming, improve mood and emotion).
- Stress and stress related conditions.
- Uplifting.

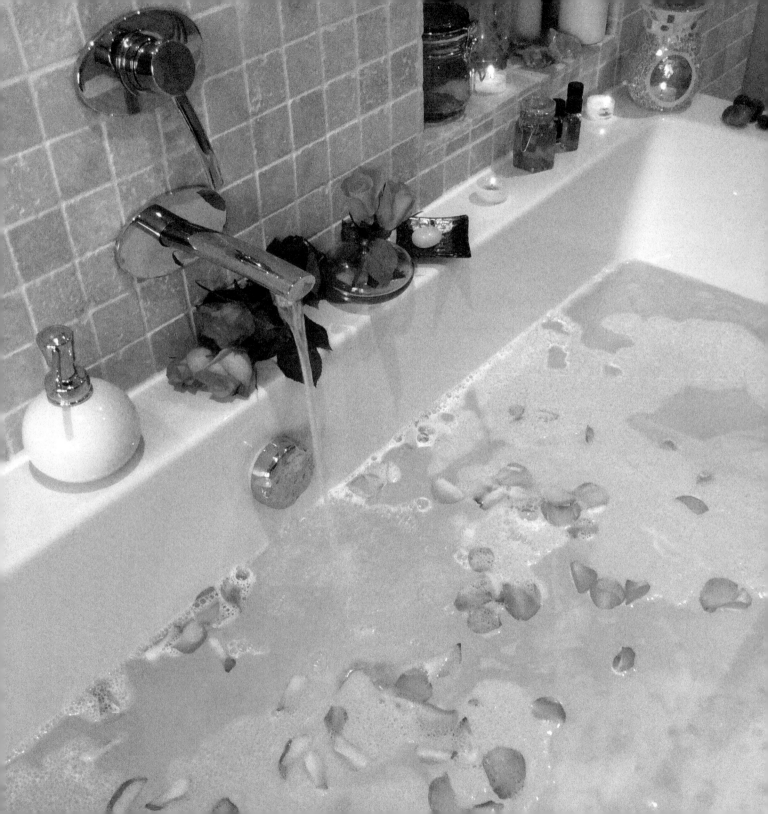

Baths

Therapeutic

Fill bath with water, then, just before getting in, add 6 to 8 drops of essential oil or an essential oil blend dispersed in 20 ml of vegetable oil or full fat milk. Do not use essential oils neat in the bath (with the exception of tea tree and lavender). To maximize benefit, close windows and doors.

Remember, vegetable oil makes the bath slippery.

Disperse essential oils into the bath in full fat milk for children, the frail or very elderly. Do not leave children unattended in a bath.

Essential oils are usually absorbed via inhalation of odour-infused steam when applied in a bath, rather than via the epidermis (skin). Although wetting and soaking the skin with warm water may assist epidermal absorption, hot or warm baths tend to encourage perspiration (excretion) rather than absorption. Water is also 'drying' to the skin; dispensing essential oil in an oily or fatty carrier medium helps form a barrier, which may prevent essential oil irritation and reduce the 'drying' effect of water.

CAUTION: NON 'GEM' ESSENTIAL OILS THAT SHOULD NOT BE USED IN THE BATH

Basil, cinnamon, clove, peppermint, thyme

Uses:

- Relaxation.
- Stress and stress related conditions.
- Superficial skin conditions.
- Respiratory conditions, including colds and 'flu.
- Uplifting.
- Anti-depressing.
- Improve mood and emotion.
- Insomnia (bathing before bedtime).
- Calm restlessness and agitation.

Alongside essential oils and Mindfulness practice, other team players in the wellness supporting toolbox, aiding the individual maintain their locus of control of their own wellbeing, also include relaxation techniques, exercise and nutrition. For example:

Exercise and mobility

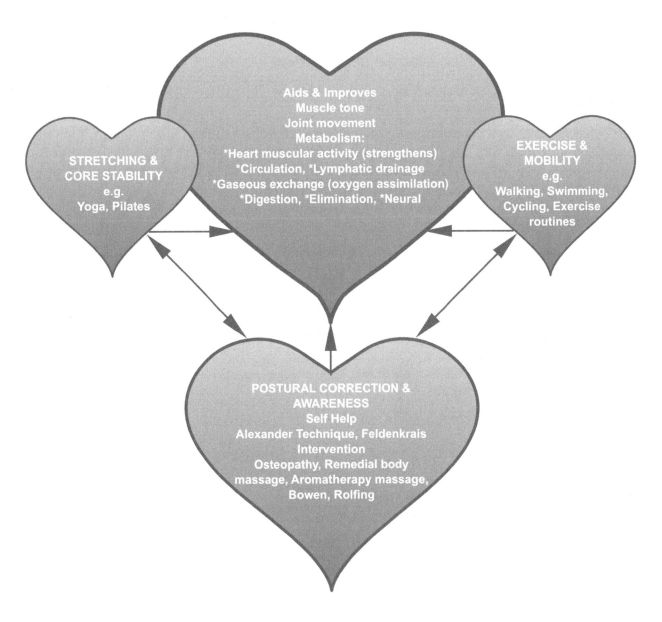

STRETCHING & CORE STABILITY
e.g.
Yoga, Pilates

Aids & Improves
Muscle tone
Joint movement
Metabolism:
*Heart muscular activity (strengthens)
*Circulation, *Lymphatic drainage
*Gaseous exchange (oxygen assimilation)
*Digestion, *Elimination, *Neural

EXERCISE & MOBILITY
e.g.
Walking, Swimming, Cycling, Exercise routines

POSTURAL CORRECTION & AWARENESS
Self Help
Alexander Technique, Feldenkrais
Intervention
Osteopathy, Remedial body massage, Aromatherapy massage, Bowen, Rolfing

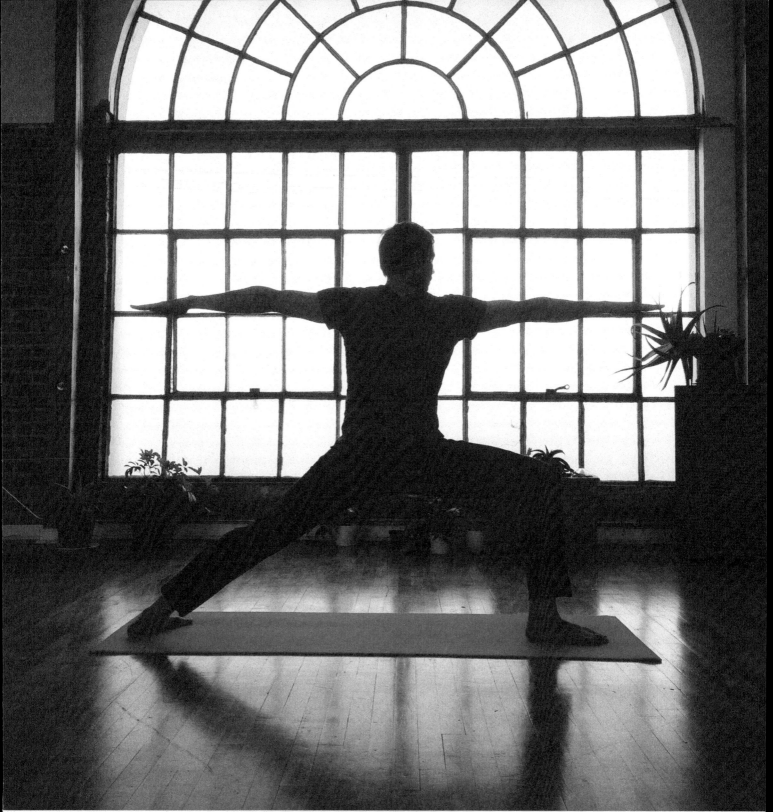

Nutritional values of food

It is advisable to eat during periods of relaxation. Do not 'eat on the go'. If you are feeling anxious, eat little and often to maintain your blood sugar levels (low blood sugar exacerbates feelings of anxiety), and include slow energy releasing carbohydrates, such as oats and other whole grains, in your diet. Do not skip meals; eat well at breakfast, moderately at lunch and suppertime (do not eat heavy meals in the evening). Drink plenty of water in between meals. Eat a varied range of fresh foods to ensure intake of vital nutrients (proteins, carbohydrates, fats, vitamins, minerals and trace elements); this range can be consumed over a week. Of course, another important factor affecting efficient assimilation of nutrients is to ENJOY YOUR FOOD. A vegetarian diet results in a greatly reduced carbon footprint (farming and food production) compared to a diet high in meat and animal products, a vegan diet even less (Burwell & Vilsick 2015). This does not mean meat should be eliminated, but eaten in moderation and sourced from ethical, environmentally friendly suppliers. The quality of the soil in which vegetables and grains are grown affects the mineral and trace element content of the plant. The following information will enable you to select foods rich in appropriate nutrients to balance your diet. The foods listed here provide macro-nutrients (protein, carbohydrate, fat, water) as well as micro-nutrients (vitamin, minerals and trace elements) and fibre required for health digestion.

A balanced diet consists of: fruit and vegetables (35%), carbohydrates: rice and grains, cereals, pasta, bread (35%), proteins: soya, pulses, meat, fish (15%), dairy: milk, cheese (10%), foods containing fats and sugars (5%).

Vitamin A

Sources: Retinoids (animal sources), fish, liver, eggs, milk (including unskimmed), butter, cheese, dairy produce. Beta-carotene (vegetable sources) soya beans, carrots, yams, sweet potatoes, pumpkin, other yellow vegetables; apricots, peaches, papaya, cantaloupe melon.
(Supports immune system, cell growth, vision)
Symptoms of deficiency: Red itchy eyes, night blindness, vision difficulties in dim light, sensitivity to bright light; dry rough skin; a predisposition to colds and infection; broken tooth enamel; kidney stones; allergies.

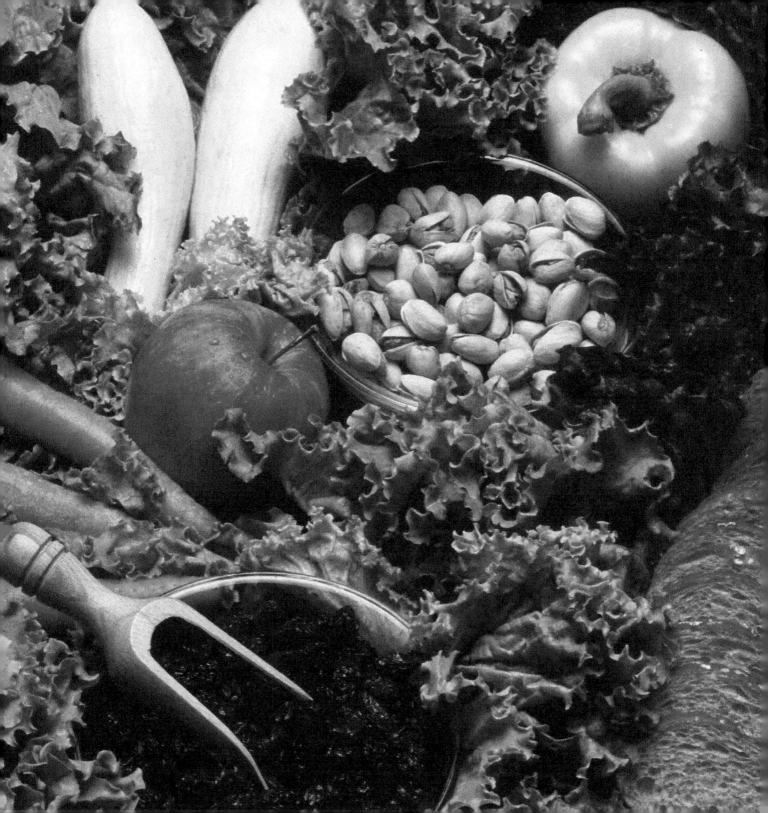

Vitamin B1 Thiamine

Sources: Liver, milk, egg yolk, legumes (beans, peas, lentils, peanuts etc.), rice, bran and raw germ of cereals, brewers yeast, molasses, green leafy and yellow vegetables, fruit.

(Rapidly destroyed by heat; aids assimilation of carbohydrates, helps convert blood sugar into energy; aids breakdown of proteins and carbohydrates, memory function, mucous membrane integrity, development of myelin sheaths and nerve function)

Symptoms of deficiency: Nervous disorders: neurosis, neurasthenia (nervous exhaustion), irritability, sensitivity to noise, loss of morale, fear, anxiety, confusion; low thyroid function; appetite loss; heart palpitations.

Vitamin B2 Riboflavin

Sources: Liver, fish roe, eggs, milk and dairy produce, brewer's yeast, green leafy vegetables.

(Concerned with carbohydrate and protein metabolism, skin development and function, blood cells and lining of intestinal tract)

Symptoms of deficiency: Mouth and lip lesions, tongue inflammation, sensation of sand in eyes, red itchy eyes, cataracts; scaly skin on face, impairment of red blood cell formation leading to anaemia and heart disease; dental problems; congenital birth defects.

Vitamin B3 Niacin

Sources: Liver, fish, eggs, brewer's yeast, raw wheat germ, peanut butter, avocados, dried fruits e.g. dates, figs, prunes.

(Associated with energy releasing in cells; aids body to utilize carbohydrates, proteins, fatty acids to create energy; works with other B Vitamins to convert macronutrients into energy)

Symptoms of deficiency: Pellagra (disease that may result in scaly skin, diarrhoea, mental disorders); indigestion, fatigue, mouth disorders, loss of sense of humour, headaches, depression, dementia, schizophrenia.

Vitamin B5 Pantothenic acid

Sources: Meat, organ meat (liver, kidney), cods roe, royal jelly, raw wheat germ, whole grains, beans, brewer's yeast, molasses, nuts.

(Associated with amino acid metabolism; aids efficient utilization of carbohydrates, proteins and lipids, skin regeneration)

Symptoms of deficiency: Mental stress, irritability, depression, hypoglycaemia, allergies, arthritis, gastric conditions – ulcers, indigestion and constipation, fatigue, greying hair, skin disorders.

Vitamin B6 Pyridoxine

Sources: Liver, kidney, eggs, milk, peas, beans, soya beans, brewer's yeast, raw wheat germ, molasses, cabbage.
(Associated with supporting proper function of carbohydrates, lipids and amino acid metabolism, the production of antibodies)
Symptoms of deficiency: Skin striations, linear nail ridges, inability to tan, sensitive to sun, tongue inflammation, cracks around lips, numbness of hands and feet, convulsions in children, depression, tremors and seizures (as in Parkinsonism and epilepsy), hypoglycaemia, diabetes, appetite loss, high cholesterol, kidney stones, arthritis, allergies, anaemia, oedema, poor dream recall.

Vitamin B12 Cyabaocobalamin

Sources: Liver, kidney, meat, eggs, dairy products, fermented liquors, yeast.
(Essential for maintenance of myelin, the nervous system and spinal cord nerves, production of elements of DNA, red blood cells, regeneration of bone marrow and lining of the gastrointestinal and respiratory tract, and melatonin production)
Symptoms of deficiency: Severe - pernicious anaemia; Mild - sore tongue, shortness of breath, heart palpitations, apathy, weakness, loss of co-ordination, impaired memory, senile dementia, sharp mood swings.

Vitamin B15 Pangamic acid

Sources: Brewer's yeast, brown rice, whole grains, pumpkin, sesame seeds.
(Antioxidant, stimulates cellular respiration and prevents cellular oxidization, aids the formation of amino acids, enhances liver function, mildly stimulant to endocrine and nervous system)
Symptoms of deficiency: Reduced oxygenation of cells, leading to fatigue, low levels of fitness, premature aging, heart disease, glandular and nervous conditions.

PABA Para-Amino Benzoic Acid B Vitamin

Sources: Liver, kidney, brewer's yeast, whole grains, raw wheat germ, molasses.
(Aids utilization of pantothenic acid, formation of red blood cells, coenzyme in metabolism and utilsation of protein, anti-oxidant; can block skin penetration of ultraviolet light, aids skin pigmentation)
Symptoms of deficiency: Eczema, wrinkles, pigmentation loss, fatigue, irritability, depression, senility, arthritis, bursitis, gastric disorders.

Folic Acid, Folate, Vitamin B9

Sources: Liver, kidney, egg yolk, torula yeast, beans, green leafy vegetables, carrots, cantaloupe melons, pumpkin, avocados.

(Aids healthy development of cells, key to the synthesis of nucleic acid)
Symptoms of deficiency: Megaloblastic anaemia, depression, psychosis, epileptic fits, lack of appetite, sore tongue, digestive disturbances.

Biotin B Vitamin (also known as Vitamin H)

Sources: Liver, egg yolk, milk, nuts, brewer's yeast, brown rice, fruits, tomatoes.
(Coenzyme, synthesised by microbes in intestine; associated with metabolism of carbohydrates; supports healthy skin, digestive tract, nerves, metabolism, cell formation and regeneration)
Symptoms of deficiency: Eczema, dermatitis, lack of appetite, fatigue, muscle aches and pains.

Choline

Sources: Brain, liver, egg yolk, brewer's yeast, raw wheat germ, green leafy vegetables.
(Made in the liver from components in the foods above; supports nervous system)
Symptoms of deficiency: Fatty degeneration of liver, nephritis (kidney disease), gallstones, intolerance of fats (gallbladder syndrome), nerve-muscle diseases, high cholesterol, atherosclerosis, hypertension.

Inositol

Sources: Liver, kidney, brain, brewer's yeast, wheat germ, molasses, peanut butter, cantaloupe melons.
(Made from glucose and found in foods above as myo-inositol; present in all living cells)
Symptoms of deficiency: Hypertension, high cholesterol levels, atherosclerosis, dermatitis, constipation, hair loss. NOTE: diabetics, alcohol and coffee drinkers over excrete inositol and therefore need supplements to prevent deficiency.

Vitamin C Ascorbic acid

Sources: Whole citrus fruits and juices (fresh), blackcurrants, elderberries, rosehips, peppers, broccoli, tomatoes, cabbage, green leafy vegetables, melons, yams, potatoes (raw to semi-cooked)
(Anti oxidant; keeps cholesterol in blood stream from oxidizing; associated with metabolism of protein; important factor in collagen production; easily damaged by heat)
Symptoms of deficiency: Susceptibility to colds, infections and allergies, bleeding or inflamed gums, defective teeth; broken capillaries and sub skin haemorrhages, strokes, anaemia, skin wrinkles, loss of appetite, fatigue, nervousness, anxiety, depression, impaired healing of wounds.

Vitamin D

Sources: Fish liver oil, sardines, herring, salmon, tuna, fortified milk, eggs, butter, cheese.
(Metabolized via sun exposure on skin, and foods above; regulates calcium and phosphorus metabolism, important factor for healthy bones and teeth)
Symptoms of deficiency: Soft and porous bones and teeth, leading to rickets and tooth decay, osteoporosis; fatigue, arthritis, myopia (short sightedness)

Vitamin E

Sources: Egg yolk, butter, milk, nuts, soya beans, whole grains and cereals. Raw wheat germ and wheat germ oil, vegetable oils, leafy green vegetables.
(Antioxidant, important for cell membrane integrity, prevents catabolism of polyunsaturated fats, protects artery walls, and myelin sheaths surrounding nerves)
Symptoms of deficiency: Fatigue, premature aging, infertility, sterility, miscarriage, muscular dystrophy, haemolytic anaemia, coronary heart disease, thrombosis, swollen and inflamed veins, lameness due to poor circulation (nephritis), degeneration of sex glands (testes, prostate), poor healing of wounds and burns.

Vitamin K

Sources: Liver, fish, fish liver oil, egg yolk, yoghurt, buttermilk, alfalfa, green leafy vegetables, kelp, safflower and soya bean oil.
(Aids blood clotting/coagulation, synthesis of proteins, binds calcium in bones; directly involved in photosynthesis)
Symptoms of deficiency: Causes delayed blood clotting, haemorrhages, lack of blood platelets. Deficiency usually caused by defect in metabolism or a malfunction of the liver, colitis or coeliac disease. Coeliac disease is caused by intestinal intolerance to gluten, a protein found in wheat, rye and barley.

Vitamin P Prolintane or Flavanoids

Sources: Citrus fruits (especially the pith and rind), grapes, plums, blackcurrants, apricots, buckwheat leaves, cherries, rose hips.
(Produced as a by-product of plant metabolism; reduces blood sugar, lipids, improves insulin resistance; anti inflammatory; aids absorption of iron)
Symptoms of deficiency: Bruising.

Calcium (Ca)

Sources: Some fish, particularly tinned fish, milk, cheese, dairy products, sesame seeds and tahini, soybeans, peanuts, walnuts, sunflower seeds, honey, molasses, green leafy vegetables.
(Associated with Vitamin D and phosphorus in the hardening of bones and teeth; involved

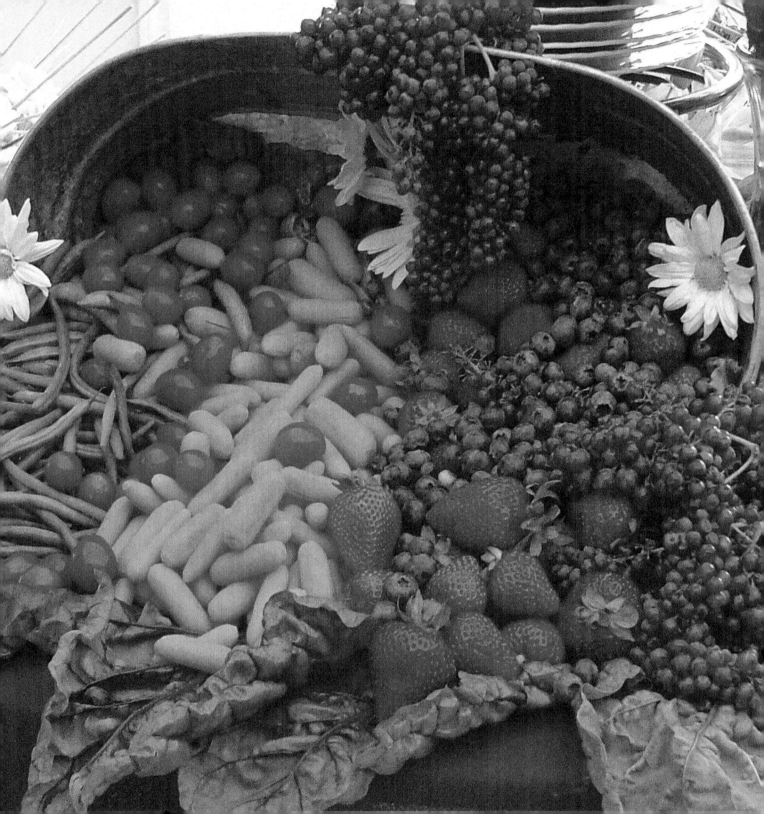

in the coagulation of blood and action of muscle contraction)
Symptoms of deficiency: Porous and brittle bones, fractures, tooth decay, rickets, nervousness, muscle aches, leg cramps, teeth grinding, skin disorders, loss of pigmentation, cold sores, mouth blisters, excessive menstrual flow, impaired growth.

Phosphorus (P)

Sources: Meat, liver, kidney, fish, eggs, cheese, nuts and seeds, whole grains, raw wheat germ, oatmeal.
(Associated with calcium and Vitamin D in hardening of bones and teeth; helps maintain the constant composition of the body fluids)
Symptoms of deficiency: Weak bones and teeth, rickets, gum infection and bleeding, arthritis, loss of appetite, muscle weakness.

Potassium (K)

Sources: Citrus fruits, green leafy vegetables, bananas, potatoes, tomatoes, pineapple, avocados, nuts (widely distributed in all foods)
(Involved in intracellular activity; contraction of muscles; transmission of nerve impulses; maintenance of the electrolyte balance in the body)
Symptoms of deficiency: Oedema, hypertension, irregular heartbeat, nervousness, fatigue, arthritis.

Sodium (Na)

Sources: Meat, shell fish, eggs, milk, artificially enriched bread, sea salt, soy sauce, tamari, kelp, beets, carrots, chard and dandelion greens.
(Works with potassium ions to build up charges on cell membrane assisting transmission of nerve impulses)
Symptoms of deficiency: Intestinal gas, weight loss, muscle wasting, fatigue, dehydration
NOTE: deficiencies are very uncommon but can be caused by excessive perspiration.

Magnesium (Mg)

Sources: Nuts (especially almonds), seeds, wheat germ, yellow corn, whole grains (especially brown rice, millet), beans, peas, figs, lemons, grapefruits, apples, green leafy vegetables, coffee, natural supplement – dolomite.
(Required for over 300 biochemical reactions of the body; supports growth and maintenance of bones, heart, nerve and muscle function, immune system)
Symptoms of deficiency: Irregular heart beat and heart attacks, 'jumpy nerves', weak muscles, convulsions and seizures, prostrate enlargement, fatigue, bedwetting, kidney stones.

Sulphur (S)

Sources: A nonmetallic mineral, abundant in nature and present in every animal and plant cell. Present in four amino acids, thiamine and biotin (B Vitamins)
(Supports enzyme reactions and protein synthesis, collagen formation, cell respiration; necessary for maintenance of hair, nails, skin)
Symptoms of deficiency: Arthritis, dry hair, brittle nails and rough skin.

Iron (Fe)

Sources: Liver, kidney, beef, raw clams, oysters, egg yolk, dried beans, oatmeal, molasses, dried peaches, raisins, prunes, green leafy vegetables.
(A vital mineral that aids transportation of oxygen around body and is involved in conversion of blood-sugar into energy. A component of haemoglobin – red blood cells. Aids maintenance of healthy hair, skin, nails)
Symptoms of deficiency: Iron deficiency – anaemia, pallor, weakness, shortness of breath, brittle nails.

Zinc (Zn)

Sources: Meat, fish, raw oysters, egg yolks, milk, dried legumes, whole grains, raw wheat germ, brewer's yeast, pumpkin seeds, sunflower seeds, ground mustard seeds, mushrooms.
(Antioxidant; protects against aging of skin and muscles; supports immune system; supports cell division and growth; vital for brain activity during detection of taste and smell; vital for healthy vision)
Symptoms of deficiency: Prostate trouble, sterility, delayed sexual maturation, menstrual irregularities, retarded growth and dwarfism, birth defects such as mental retardation and slow learning, susceptibility to infections and poor wound healing, joint pains, artherosclerosis and poor circulation, fatigue, lack of appetite, loss of sense of taste and smell, susceptibility to diabetes, allergies, acne, stretch marks, de-pigmentation (white spots) of nails, offensive perspiration.

Copper (Cu)

Sources: Liver, kidney, sea foods, especially shell fish, soybeans, legumes (beans, lentils), whole grain especially whole wheat and rye, molasses, chocolate, peanuts, pecans, prunes, kale, apples.
(Necessary for producing and storing iron and for healthy function of organs and metabolism; necessary for proper growth, development and maintenance of bone, connective tissue, brain, heart; involved in formation of red blood cells, synthesis and release of life-sustaining proteins and enzymes)

Symptoms of deficiency: Anaemia, fatigue, shortness of breath, skin de-pigmentation.

Manganese (Mn)

Sources: Nuts, pumpkin seeds, whole grains, whole wheat, oats, peas, cloves, ginger, tea leaves, green leafy vegetables, especially spinach, watercress, beetroot, peppermint, strawberries, blackberries, bananas, molasses.

(Necessary for development, metabolism; anti-oxidant; stored in bones, liver and kidneys)

Symptoms of deficiency: Low tolerance to carbohydrates, skeletal abnormalities (legs too short or long) loss of muscle condition, convulsions.

Chromium (Cr)

Sources: Meat, eggs, shell fish, clams, brewer's yeast, molasses, raw wheat germ, rice bran, broccoli, garlic, basil, apples, bananas, green beans.

(Aids balance of blood-sugar by supporting body's use of insulin; aid metabolism and storage of carbohydrates, fat and protein)

Symptoms of deficiency: Fatigue, slow growth, obesity, hypertension, high cholesterol levels, impaired glucose metabolism, diabetes.

Iodine (I)

Sources: Shell fish, kelp, seaweeds, onions, strawberries, milk, yogurt, eggs,sea salt.

(Constituent of thyroxine and trilodothyronine; has nutritional relationship with selenium; necessary for healthy function of gastric mucosa, salivary glands, arterial walls, thymus, epidermis, choroid plexus, cerebrospinal fluid, breasts during lactation)

Symptoms of deficiency: Goitre – characterised by swelling of the thyroid gland in the lower neck; hypothyroidism – symptoms include obesity, dry hair, rapid pulse, heart palpitations, a cold body, constipation, weakness, excessive menstruation, nervousness, low resistance to colds and infections, irritability.

Selenium (Se)

Sources: Liver, fish – tuna, mackerel, halibut, herring; shell fish – oysters, scallops, lobster, butter, brazil nuts, sunflower seeds, raw wheat germ, brewer's yeast, garlic, onions, whole grains. Selenium is destroyed when foods are processed – a variety of whole, unprocessed foods provides best source of dietary selenium.

(Anti-oxidant, especially when combined with Vitamin E; catalyst for production of active thyroid hormone; proper function of immune system; required for sperm motility)

Symptoms of deficiency: Fatigue, susceptibility to infections and disease, premature aging, predisposition to cancer, low sex drive, mood swings.

Fluorine (Fl)

Sources: Seafood, cheese, kelp, fluoridated drinking water, tea, small amounts naturally occur in water, air, plants, animals.

(Essential for mineralisation of bones and formation of dental enamel; present in bones, teeth, thyroid gland, skin)

Symptoms of deficiency: Demineralisation of bones and teeth, wrinkled skin, lowered resistance to colds and infections, low energy levels.

Molybdenum (Mo)

Sources: Organ meat, milk, cheese, eggs, legumes (lentils, beans, peas), nuts, seeds, whole grain cereals, dark green leafy vegetables, green beans, cucumber.

(Stored in the liver, kidneys, glands, bones, tooth enamel; plays important role in normal body functions – protecting cells, creating energy, supporting liver and kidneys to remove waste products; aids in the metabolism of fats and carbohydrates, breakdown of certain amino acids)

Symptoms of deficiency: Predisposition to tooth decay, anaemia, oesophalgeal cancer, lowered sexual potency (men)

Germanium (Ge)

Sources: Trace amounts in most foods. Richer amounts in ginseng, garlic, aloe vera, comfrey, broccoli, celery, mushrooms, rhubarb, tomato juice.

(Acts against inflammation; balances/regulates body's ions and removes excess positive ions; strengthens immune system, improves blood circulation, raises oxygen levels, speeds up metabolism of body cells, removes harmful toxins, reduces cholesterol levels)

Symptoms of deficiency: Increased susceptibility to the degenerative diseases associated with aging, infection and immune disorders, heart disease, high cholesterol, arthritis, osteoporosis.

Boron (B)

Sources: Fruits – apples, peaches, oranges, red grapes, pears, plums, currents, kiwis, sultanas, dates, tomatoes. Vegetables – avocado, olives, onion, soybeans, chickpeas, red kidney beans, borlotti beans, lentils, hazel nuts, nutritional supplements.

(Affects the way the body utilizes other minerals – magnesium, phosphorus; increases oestrogen levels in post – menopausal women)

Symptoms of deficiency: Calcium loss, bone demineralisation, arthritis, low oestrogen levels in menopause, reduced growth. Abnormal metabolism of calcium and magnesium.

Protein

Protein is the collective label applied to identify amino acids. Amino acids are organic compounds composed of amine (-NH2) and carboxylic acid (-COOH) with additional amino acid specific carbon 'side chains' which are attached to a main chain or 'backbone'. Proteins form the second largest component of muscle cells and body tissues; water comprises the largest. There are around 500 known amino acids. However, just twenty-two standard amino acids are required for proper function of the body; nine are vital because they cannot be created from other compounds by the body so they must be eaten and absorbed. There are two types of protein: complete (first class) and incomplete (second class). Complete proteins contain all the required amino acids in one food source that are necessary to maintain health. Incomplete proteins, mainly found in vegetables, do not. Incomplete proteins can be combined to provide a range of amino acids that ultimately create a complete protein (these can be consumed in different meals during the day, they do not need to all be present in one meal). Grains such as wheat, rice and corn, when combined with legumes such as beans, peas and lentils, collectively provide sufficient amino acids to form a whole protein; similarly, hummus and pitta bread, peanut butter and whole wheat bread, rice and dhal (lentils) etc.

Amino acids required by the body for proper function

Essential
(cannot be made within the body)

- Histidine
- Isoleucine
- Leucine
- Lysine
- Methionine
- Phenylalanine
- Threonine
- Tryptophan
- Valine

Non-essential
(*essential in some circumstances, e.g. children to support growth)

- Alanine
- Arginine*
- Asparagine
- Aspartic acid
- Cysteine*
- Glutamic acid
- Glutamine*
- Glycine
- Pyrrolysine*
- Proline*
- Selenocysteine*
- Serine*
- Tyrosine*

Protein type	Food sources which supply protein	Required by the body for:
Complete (first class)	**Animal sources** Meat, fish, eggs, milk, cheese and other milk products except butter **Plant sources** Quinoa, buckwheat, hempseed, chia, soy **Combined vegetable sources** Grains (rice, wheat, corn) + legumes (beans, peas, lentils) Spirulina + grains + nuts	**Cells**: nucleoproteins found in nucleus of every cell **Enzymes**: break down food for absorption, nutrient absorption and waste removal in cells; growth, development, movement reproduction **Haemoglobin:** proteins + iron carry oxygen around the body **Myoglobin** and **elastin**: found in muscle fibres **Bones**: mainly comprise of protein (+ calcium, magnesium, phosphate) **Hormones:** regulation of metabolism **Antibodies**: immunity **Keratin:** to form nails and hair

Incomplete (second class)	Vegetables which contain amino acids (protein) Soy beans, lentils, black beans, chick peas, chai seeds, tofu, pumpkin seeds, sunflower seeds, rolled oats, buckwheat, green peas, almond butter, peanut butter, almonds and other nuts, quinoa, millet, rye grains, wheat, brown rice, corn, flax seeds, coconut, broccoli, spinach, spirulina, kale, romaine lettuce	Signs and Symptoms of Deficiency Oedema, weight loss, thinning or brittle hair, ridges in nails, pale skin, skin rashes, general weakness, slow healing, difficulty sleeping, headaches, fainting Other symptoms: crankiness, moodiness, depression, anxiety, lack of energy, no desire to do things
Daily requirement	Infants aged 1 to 3 years old 13g Children aged 4 to 8 years old 19g Children aged 9 to 13 years old 34g	Girls aged 14 to 18 years old 46g Boys aged 14 to 18 years old 52g Women aged 19 years + 46g Men aged 19 years + 56g

Perfume 'Notes'		
Top	**Middle**	**Base**
Cajeput (*Melaleuca cajeputii*)	**Carrot Seed** (*Daucus carota*)	**Frankincense (Olibanum)** (*Boswellia carterii*)
Galbanum (*Ferula galbaniflua*)	**Chamomile German** (*Matricaria recutita*)	**Patchouli** (*Pogostemon cablin* Benth.)
Mandarin (*Citrus reticulata*)	**Chamomile Roman** (*Chamaemelum nobile; Anthemis nobilis*)	**Rose Otto*** (*Rosa x centifolia* L. *Rosa damascene* Mil. spp.)
Petitgrain (*Citrus amara; Citrus aurantium* Linn)	**Cypress** (*Cupressus sempervirens*)	**Spikenard (Nard)** (*Nardostachys jatamansi* D.C. *Nardostachys grandiflora* D.C.)
Tea Tree (*Melaleuca alternifolia Cheel*)	**Geranium** (*Pelargonium graveolens roseum; Pelargonium roseum asperum L'Herit.* spp)	**Vetivert** (*Vetiveria zizanoides* L. Stapf.)
	Lavender (*Lavandula angustifolia* Mill. (*Lavandula vera* D.C. spp.)	
	Lavender Spike (*Lavandula latifolia*)	

*Distilled Rose Otto essential oil is very expensive to purchase and, therefore, often adulterated. Rose absolute is produced by solvent extraction and contains residue of the solvent and other 'washout' material used; Rose absolute is less expensive, however, and although not classed as a 'pure' essential oil, nonetheless, procures similar hedonistic effects. Rose Geranium (Pelargonium graveolens roseum) has similar properties to Rose essential oil and may be used as a less expensive substitute in some instances.

Products containing essential oils

Alcohol

Air-fresheners

Animal feed

Antiseptics

Baked goods

Beverages (earl grey tea, jasmine and rose tea, herbal teas)

Candle making

Confectionary

Contact lenses

Convenience foods

Cosmetics and toiletries

Cough syrups

Dentistry products

Detergents

Disinfectants

Fabric conditioner

Food and drink flavouring

Food colouring

Gargles

Glue / adhesives

Household products

Ice cream

Insect repellants / insecticides

Lotions, creams

Meat products

Mouthwash

Nasal sprays

Ointments

Paint

Paper

Perfumery (eau-de-cologne)

aftershave)

Pharmaceuticals

Pizzas

Preservatives

Printing ink

Rubber manufacturing

Soaps

Soap Powder

Soft drinks

Stomachic / laxatives

Tinned food

Textile products

Throat lozenges

Tobacco

Toothpaste

Veterinary products

Reference and Bibliography

- Alexander, M (2000 How Theories of Motivation Apply to Olfactory Aromatherapy: International Journal of Aromatherapy: Harcourt Publishers: vol 16 nos. 3 / 4: p 196-210

- Beauregard, M. (2007) Mind does really matter: Evidence from Neuro-imaging studies of emotional self-regulation, psychotherapy, and placebo effect: Progress in Neurobiology 81: Elservier: p 218-236

- Beshara, M. C.; Giddings, D. (2002) Use of Plant essential oils in Treating Agitation in a Dementia Unit; International Journal of Aromatherapy: Churchill Livingston Harcourt Publishers: vol 12 not 4: p 207-212

- Bible: http://www.kingjamesbibleonline.org/book.php?book=Jeremiah&chapter=6&verse=20 : sourced 2014

- Bryan-Jefferies (2005) Person-Centred Counselling Supervision: Radcliffe Publishing: p 14, 15

- Buchbauer et al (1992) Fragrance Compounds and Essential Oils with Sedative Effects upon Inhalation: Journal of Pharmaceutical Science: vol. 82 no. 6 June 1993: p 661

- Burch, V. (2010) The mindful way to well being: The Breathworks Approach: http://www.breathworks-mindfulness.org.uk/PDF/Breathworks_mindfulness_article_Jan_2010.pdf (sourced 2014)

- Burwell, S. M.: Vilsak, T. J. (2105) USDA Scientific Report of the Dietary Guidelines Advisory Committee: http://www.health.gov/dietaryguidelines/2015-scientific-report/PDFs/

- Busse, D.; Kudella, P.; Gruning, N-M; Gisselmann, G.; Stander, S.; Luger, T.; Jacobson, F.; Steinstraber, L.; Paus, R.; Gkogkolou, P.; Bohm, M.; Hatt, H.; Benecke, H. (2014) A Synthetic Sandalwood Odorant Induces Wound Healing Process in Human Keratinocytes via Olfactory Receptor OR2AT4: Journal of Investigative Dermatology vol 134 p 2823-2832: http://www.nature.com/jid/journal/v134/n11/abs/jid2014273a.html

- Carmody, J. (2009) Evolving Conceptions of Mindfulness in Clinical Settings: Journal of Psychotherapy: An International Quarterly: vol 23 no 3 p 272

- Chambers R.; Gullone, E.; Allen, N. B. (2009) Mindful emotion regulation An Integrative review: Clinical Psychology Review 29: p 560-567 p 562
- Clarkson, P. (1999) Gestalt Counselling in Action (2nd ed.); Sage Publications, London
- Cordon, L. S.; Brown, K. W.; Gibson, P. R.: (2009) The Role of Mindfulness Based Stress Reduction on Perceived Stress: Preliminary Evidence for the Moderating Role of Attachment Style: Journal of Cognitive Psychotherapy: An International Quarterly: vol 23 no 3
- Damian, 1995; Damian, P.; Damian, K. (1995) Scent & Psyche: Using Essential Oils for Physical and Emotional Well-being: Healing Arts Press: Rochester, Vermont; p 94, 141-165
- Davidson, J. L. (2002) Aromatherapy and Work-Related Stress: International Journal of Aromatherapy: Harcourt Publishers: vol 12 no 3: p 145-151
- Fromm, E. (1998) The Art of Listening: Constable London: p 39, 95 89)
- Gabriel, L. (2005) Speaking the Unspeakable: Routledge:
- Gattefosse, R-M (1995) Aromatherapy (first published in 1935): The CW Daniel Co Ltd: Saffron Walden
- Godfrey, H (2005) Counselling: A Journey in Experiential Learning; Aromatherapy Times (International quarterly journal of the IFA) Volume 1 no. 65 pg 10-12
- Godfrey, H. (2002) Counselling Skills: An Inseparable Aspect of Therapeutic Relationships; Aromatherapy Times (International quarterly journal of the IFA) Volume 1 no. 55 pg 28-31
- Godfrey, H. (2009) Essential Oils: Complementary Treatment for Attention Deficit Hyperactive Disorder: International Journal of Clinical Aromatherapy: Essential Oil Resource Consultants SARL: France: vol 6 issue 1: p14-22
- Godfrey, H. (2011) Aromatherapy: Purely Simply, Effectively: Boundaries of Professional Practice (International Journal of Clinical Aromatherapy – publish date tbc)
- Goldin, P PhD; Ramel, W. PhD; Gross, J. PhD (2009) Mindfulness Meditation Training and Self-Referential Processing in Social Anxiety Disorder: Behavioural and Neural Effects: Journal of Cognitive Psychotherapy: An International Quarterly: vol 23 no 3
- Griffin, C. A.; kafadar, K. A.; Pavlath, G. K. (2009) MOR23 promotes muscle regeneration and regulates cell adhesion and migration; US National Library of Medicine, National Institute of Health PubMed: http://www.ncbi.nlm.nih.gov/pmc/articles/PMC2780437/

- Gunaratana, B. H. (2009) Beyond Mindfulness: in plain English: Wisdom Publications, Boston: p 2, 17, 33, 34
- Halden, P (2003) An Exploration of the effectiveness of a work based initiative to improve the working lives of staff: Submission for award of MSc in Practitioner research, Faculty of Community Studies, Law and Education, Manchester Metropolitan University, England;
  http://www.mmu.ac.uk/study/postgraduate/research/2011
- Hanh T. N. (1991) The Miracle of Mindfulness: Ryder, London
- Hawkins, P.; Shohet, R. (2004) Approaches to the Supervision of Cousellors: found in Dryden, W.; Thorne, B. (2004) Training and Supervision for Counselling in Action: Sage Publications
- Hawkins, P.; Shohet, R. (2006) Supervision in the Helping Professions: Open University Press: p 6, 81
- Holzel, B. K.; Caromody, J.; Vangel, M.; Congleton, C; Yerramset, S. M. (2011) Mindfulness Practice leads to increases in regional brain gray matter density: Psychiatry Research: Neuro-imaging 191 36-43 www.elservier.com
  http://www.academia.edu/7872565/Medicinal_Plants_in_The_Quran
- Imberger et al (1993) Effects of Essential Oils on Human Attention Progresses: International Symposium On Essential Oils, Berlin
- Kabat-Zinn, J (2004) Coming To Our Senses: a conversation with Jon Kabat-Zinn: http://www.inquiringmind.com/Articles/JonKabat.html
- Kabat-Zinn, J. (2002) At Home in Our Bodies:
  http://www.bemindful.org/kabatzinnart.htm
- Kutz, L.;Borysenko, J.; Benson, H. (1985) Meditation and Psychotherapy: a rationale for the integration of dynamic psychotherapy, the relaxation response, and mindfulness meditation: American Journal of Psychiatry; 142 1-8: (found in Mace C. (2008) Mindfulness and Mental Health: Therapy, Theory and Science: Routledge, London)
- Mace, C. (2008) Mindfulness and Mental Health: Therapy, Theory and Science: Routledge, London: p 5, 6, 73, 74
- Mackenzie, C. S.; Poulin, M. A.; Seidand-Carlson, R. (2006) A Brief Minfulness Based Stress Reduction Intervention for Nurses and Nurse Aides: Applied Nursing Research 19 p 105-109
- Mearns, D.; Thorne B. (2000. (2000) Person Centred Therapy Today: : p 1-16
- Mearns, D.; Thorne, B. (1999) Person-Centred Counselling in Action: Sage Publications, London

- Mehta, P. D. (1989) Holistic Consciousness: Reflections of the Destiny of Humanity: Element Books, Shaftsbury: p 36

- Muhammad, A. (sourced 2014) Medicinal Flora in Holy Quran: http://www.academia.edu/7872565/Medicinal_Plants_in_The_Quran

- National Institute for Mental Health (2014) Transforming the understanding and treatment of mental illness: Mental Health Medications:

  http://www.nimh.nih.gov/health/publications/mental-health-medications/index.shtml

- Ong, J.: Sholtes, D. (2010) A Mindfulness-Based Approach to the Treatment of Insomnia: Journal of Clinic Psychology:

- Pipe, T. B.; Pendergast, D.; (2009) Nurse Leader Mindfulness Meditation Prgram for Stress Management: The Journal of Nursing Administration; vol 39 no 3 P 130-137

- Pluznick, J. L.; Zou, D-J.; Zhang, X.; Yan, Q.; Rodriguez-Gil, D. J.; Eisner, C.; Wells, E.; Greer, C. A.; Wang, T.; Firestein, S.; Schnermann, J.; Caplan, M. J. (2008) Functional expression of the olfactory signaling system in the kidney: National Academy of Science: vol 106 no 6 p 2059-2064:

  http://www.pnas.org/content/106/6/2059.full

- Prem Rawat 2011) http://tprf.org/publications

- Rinpoche, S. M. (2010) How to do Mindfulness Meditation:

  http://www.shambhalasun.com/index.php?option=content&task=view&id=2125

- Rogers, C. (1980) A Way of Being: Houghton Mifflin Company, New York: p 134

- Ryan, S. (2004) Vital Practice Stories from the Healing Arts: The Homeopathic and Supervisory Way: Sea Change: p 22

- Shapiro, S. L.; Astin, J. A.; Bishop, S. R.;Cordova M.; (2005) Mindfulness-Based Stress Reduction for Helath Care Professionals: Results From A Randomised Trial: International Journal of Stress Management: vol 12 no 2 p 164-176

- Shapiro, S. L.; Schwartz, E. R.; Santree, C. (2002) Meditation and Positive Psychology: found in Snyder, C. (2002) Handbook of Positive Psychology: Oxford University Press

- Shapiro, S. L.; Shwartz G. E. R.; Santree, C. (2002) Meditation and Positive Psychology found in Snyder, C. (2002) Handbook of Positive Psychology: Oxford University Press: p 634

- Shepherd Hanger, S. (1995) The Aromatherapy Practitioners Reference Manual: Atlantic Institute of Aromatherapy: vol 1 & 2

- Shnaubelt, K (1995) Advanced Aromatherapy: The Science of Essential Oil Therapy: Healing Arts Press

- Snyder, C.; Lopez, S. (Lopez 2007) Mindfulness, Flow, and Spirituality: In Search of

Optimal Experiences: Positive Psychology: Sage Publications

- Sorensen, J. (2001) The Hormonal Activity of Vitex Agnus Castus and its Importance in Therapy: Pre published lecture paper (forwarded by author)

- Spehr, M.; Gisselmann, G.; Poplawski, A.; Riffell, J. A.; Wetzel, C. H.; Zimmer, R. K.; Hatt, H. (2003) Indentification of a testicular odorant receptor mediating human sperm chemotaxis: US National Library of Medicine, National Institute of Health PubMed: http://www.ncbi.nlm.nih.gov/pubmed/12663925

- Stone, A. (2014) Smell Turns Up in Unexpected Places: New York Times: http://www.nytimes.com/2014/10/14/science/smell-turns-up-in-unexpected-places.html?_r=0

- Tisserand, R,; Balacs, T. (1995) Essential Oil Safety: Churchill Livingstone: Edinburgh

- Tisserand, R. (1997) The Art of Aromatherapy: CW Daniel: Saffron Walden

- Tisserand, R. (2011) roberttisserand.com/aromatherapy

- Valentine, K. (2015) Americans should consider eating less meat for environmental reasons, scientists say: http://thinkprogress.org/climate/2015/02/20/3625164/

- Valnet, J (1996) The Practice of Aromatherapy: The CW Daniel Co Ltd: Saffron Walden

- Wang, D. J. J.; Rao, H.; Korczykowski, M.; Wintering, N.; Pluto, J.; Khalso, D. S.; Newberg A. B. (2010) Cerebral blood flow changes associated with different meditation practices and perceived depth of meditation: Psychiatry Research: Neuroimaging: Elsevier www.elservier.com

- Werbach, (M.D.) M. R. (1995) Nutritional Influence on Aggressive Behaviour: Journal of Orthomolecular Medicine: vol 7 no. 1

- Williams, D. G. (2000) Lecture Notes on Essential Oils: Eve Taylor (London) Ltd

- Williams, D. G. (2006:1997) The Chemistry of Essential Oils: An Introduction for Aromatherapists, Beauticians, Retailers and Students: Michelle Press: Weymouth England

About the author

Heather studied at the University of Salford and was awarded a BSc (Joint Hon) Degree in Counselling and Complementary Medicine, and Masters Certificates in Integrated Mindfulness and Supervision of Counselling and Therapeutic Relationships. She also gained a Post Graduate Teaching Certificate (PGCE) from Bolton Institute. She worked at the College of Health and Social Care at the University of Salford for nine years fulfilling multiple roles. She was Programme Lead for the BSc Integrated Therapy in Practice and BSc Complementary Therapy in Practice Top up Degrees and Module Lead and lecturer for the Aromatherapy, Supervision and CPD, and Communication and Professional Skills Modules. She was also a personal tutor.

Heather has had a number of articles and research papers published in associated professional journals, including the International Journal of Clinical Aromatherapy (IJCA). A Fellow of the International Federation of Aromatherapists (IFA), she was Chair of Education during 2013 and supports the IFA's educational programme in an advisory capacity. Through her private practice, Heather continues to provide professional training, essential oil therapy treatments, professional supervision for therapists, professional development and introductory workshops.

This book is part of a set which will also cover stress reduction, therapeutic and historical context, botany, chemistry, production and details of essential oils.

About Magic Oxygen

Magic Oxygen Limited is a little green publishing house based in Lyme Regis, Dorset. It was founded in 2011 by Tracey and Simon West, who share an enormous passion for organic seasonal food, simple green living and advocating sustainable behaviours in local and global environments; they also share a common love of the written word.

They have published 20 titles from some outstanding authors over the last few years, including Bridport Prize winning Chris Hill and the much loved children's writer, Sue Hampton. They've also showcased exceptional talent from emerging authors; these include Connor Cadellin McKee, James Dunford Wood, Anthony Ravenwood, Izzy Robertson, Leslie Tate and more. They have several multi-disciplined authors who are also playwrights and graphic novel producers; these include Max Brandt, Mark James and Robert Windsor.

New titles are hitting the bookshelf this year from Heather Godfrey and Tony Lambert amongst others and if that weren't enough diversity, they also have self-help and environmental titles from Lilly Laine, Elizabeth J Walker and Tracey herself.

For the full range see MagicOxygen.co.uk/shop and remember, every title can be ordered from local or national bookshops, and online too (they favour small independent retailers which helps keep money in local communities). Magic Oxygen are also happy to fulfil orders - they might even have a signed edition to hand!

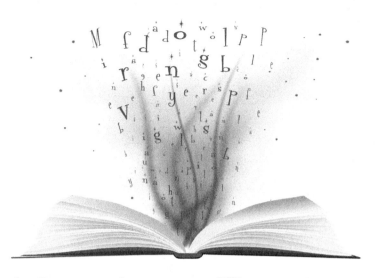

Magic Oxygen Publishing

breathing life into words

We hope you enjoyed the read!

For future literary purchases we'd like
to encourage you to buy from
your local independent bookshop.

They need your love, money and support
and all of our titles are available to order there.

#ShopLocal #BeSustainable

#MakeADifference #MOLP

The Greenest Writing Competitions in the World

Magic Oxygen have founded a series of writing contests designed to uncover literary talent from writers around the world. The main one is the Magic Oxygen Literary Prize, fondly known as MOLP, which carries a prize fund of £3,000.

In 2016 they launched the Mini-MOLPs, 5 diverse writing contests with thought provoking themes inspired by international eco-awareness events. The winners will bag 10 fabulous paperbacks from the Magic Oxygen best sellers list, plus an additional unique special prize.

These contests have a powerful environmental impact, because every single submission to MOLP and the Mini-MOLPs results in a tree being planted in Magic Oxygen's tropical Word Forest in Bore, Kenya. All entrants are sent the GPS coordinates of their trees.

This pioneering international project is carefully coordinated by forestry expert, Ru Hartwell of Community Carbon Link. He chose Kenya for the Word Forest because trees planted near the equator are the most efficient at capturing carbon from the atmosphere and keeping the planet cool. Ru specifically chose Bore because it's a remote community that has suffered greatly from deforestation. The new saplings will eventually reintroduce biodiversity, provide food, medicine and water purifiers and will create an income for the village too.

For further details and to submit entries, visit MagicOxygen.co.uk then help our reforestation project by spreading the news on social media.

Mini-MOLP April 2016:
Letter to the Planet - 350 words

Have fun deciding who your letter is from.
What have they got to say for themselves?
*Take inspiration from **Earth Day** or **National Gardening Week***

Mini-MOLP May 2016:
Eco-Flash Fiction - 250 words

Conjure up pocket-sized literary magnificence
with an uplifting green slant.
*Take inspiration from **World Biodiversity Day**
or **International Dawn Chorus Day***

Mini-MOLP June 2016:
Sonnet for the Solstice - 14 lines

Wax lyrical with a Shakespearian style sonnet and
imagine it performed at the break of day on the solstice.
*Take inspiration from **World Environment Day** or **World Oceans Day***

Mini-MOLP July 2016:
Postcard from the Park - 200 words

Pen a postcard-sized piece to anyone or anything,
with your arboreal thoughts and stories.
*Take inspiration from **National Parks Week** or **National Tree Day***

Mini-MOLP August 2016:
Last Words Monologue - 400 words

The film is about to end, the last of a species is about to die.
Write the script of their parting words.
*Take inspiration from **World Honey Bee Day** or **World Elephant Day***

CPSIA information can be obtained
at www.ICGtesting.com
Printed in the USA
FSOW04n1255210916
25230FS